100 Data Interpretation Questions in Paediatrics

Nagi Giumma Barakat MB BcH, MRCP (UK), MRCPCH, MSc (Epilepsy)

D1634733

To Lobna, Iman, Nadia, and Yasmine

100 Data Interpretation Questions in Paediatrics:

for MRCPCH/MRCP Part 2

Editor
Nagi Giumma Barakat MB BCh, MRCPCH, MSc Epilepsy
Specialist registrar
Kingston Hospital
Surrey, UK

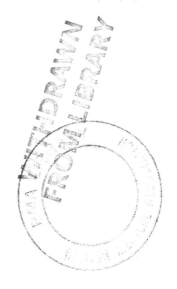

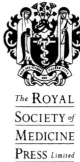

The ROYAL
SOCIETY *of*
MEDICINE
PRESS *Limited*

Contents

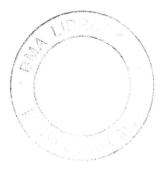

Preface

This book is designed for postgraduate candidates taking the
MRCPCH Part II exams in the UK, or the MRCP Part II paediatrics
exams in Ireland. It offers an easily accessible and very
comprehensive review of some of the most common cases and a few
of the rare ones that one may encounter. This data has been
produced after lengthy preparation as all cases are real cases which
have been collected from personal experience whilst working in
several paediatric departments over the past few years.

Nearly one third of the cases cover paediatric neurology, with five
EEGs which have not been used before. In most of the cases, there
are guidelines for which investigations to use, and how to arrive at a
positive diagnosis. I have tried to include the pathophysiology in as
many cases as possible as I find it most exciting and helpful to
understand the illness. There are a few unusual cases such as the
Aicardi syndrome which may be described to the candidate as a
failure to thrive. You may also be asked in the oral exam about
benign Rolandic epilepsy of childhood which I am sure everyone will
come across during training, or you may be asked for the differential
diagnosis of nocturnal seizures, both of which are covered in this
book.

As with examination papers, this book has been divided into ten
sections or 'papers', each of which consists of ten case presentations
and between one and four questions related to each case; answers
are given at the end of each paper. Always try to write down on paper
your answer to the questions before going on to read the answers
and explanation.

This book is a practical study aid both for the oral and clinical
examinations. Some of the answers are helpful for paediatricians to
use as guidelines for the investigation of many cases. Medical
students will learn about clinical paediatrics if they read the cases and
their explanations.

I have tried to make this book as practical and easy to read as
possible using as many interesting cases and discussions as
appropriate. I hope you enjoy using it.

NGB

Acknowledgements

Special thanks to my wife, Lobna Ali Maktari, who helped me with the editing of this book even though she is having a hard time with the twins. Also, special thanks to Dr A Winrow who encouraged me to go ahead with this book and helped me to put it together in its final layout. His comments and advice were valuable as well as his experience as an author. Thanks to all my colleagues who inspired me with many ideas and comments which had an effect on the final preparations of this book. Lastly and not least of all, good luck to all candidates for MRCPCH Part II and MRCP Part II.

Lastly, I would like to thank Professor J Aicardi, Professor Hughs, Dr G M Fenichel, Dr R J Postlethwaite and their publishers (MacKeith Press, Butterworth Heinemann and WB Saunders) for allowing me to use material from their books and journal articles.

References

Aicardi J 1998 Diseases of the Nervous system in Childhood, 2nd edn. MacKeith Press

Behrman R E, Kleigman R M, Nelson W E, Vaughan V C 1996 Nelson's Textbook of Paediatrics, 15th edn. WB Saunders, London

Campbell A G M, McIntosh N (1997) Forfar and Arneil's Textbook of Paediatrics, 5th edn. Churchill Livingstone, Edinburgh

Fenichel G M 1993 Clinical Pediatric Neurology, A sign and symptoms approach, 2nd edn. WB Saunders, London

Postlethwaite R J 1986 Clinical Paediatric Nephrology, lst edn. IOP Publishing Ltd

Various journals include: Archives of Disease in Childhood, Current Paediatrics, European Journal of Paediatric Neurology

Abbreviations

AA	Amino acids
AAFB	Alcohol and acid-fast bacilli
ABG	Arterial blood gas
ADH	Antidiuretic hormone
Alb	Albumin
Alk.ph	Alkaline phosphatase
αGT	Alpha glutamic transaminase
ALT	Alanine aminotransferase
ANA	Anti-nuclear antibodies
AO	Aorta
AR	Autosomal recessive
ASD	Atrial septal defect
ASOT	Anti-streptolysin-O-titres
AST	Aspartate aminotransferase
AXR	Abdominal X-ray
BCG	Bacillus Calmette–Guerin
Be	Base excess
Bili	Bilirubin
BMD	Bone metabolic disease
BPD	Broncho-pulmonary dysplasia
BT	Bleeding time
C3	Complement
CH50	Cytochrome 50
CK	Creatinine kinase
Cl	Chloride
CO_2	Carbon dioxide
Cr	Creatinine
CRP	C reactive protein
CT	Computerized tomography
CXR	Chest X-ray
DCT	Direct Coombs' test
DHA	Dehydroepiandrosterone
DMSA	Dimercaptosuccinic acid
DNA	Deoxyribonucleic acid
DTPA	Diethylene triamine penta-acetic acid
Echo	Echocardiograph
ELSCS	Elective lower segmental caesarean section
EMG	Electromyography
ERG	Electro-retinography
ETT	Endotracheal tube
Fib	Fibrinogen
FSH	Follicular stimulating hormone
FVC	Forced vital capacity
GFR	Glomerular filtration rate
GH	Growth hormone
Glu	Glucose

GN	Glomerulonephritis
GOR	Gastro-oesophageal reflux
Hb	Haemoglobin
HbF	Fetal haemoglobin
HbSS	Sickle cell disease
HCO_3	Bicarbonate
Hct	Haematocrit
HD	Hodgkin's disease
HMD	Hyaline membrane disease
HR	Heart rate
HVA	Homovanillic acid
Ig	Immunoglobulin
IRT	Immunoreactive trypsin
IVC	Inferior vena cava
IVH	Intraventricular haemorrhage
IVIG	Intravenous immunoglobulin
KPTT	Kaolin partial thromboplastin time
LA	Left atrium
LBBB	Left bundle branch block
LFT	Liver function test
LH	Luteinising hormone
LV	Left ventricle
MAG3	Mercapto acetyl triglycine
MAP	Mean arterial pressure
MCHC	Mean corpuscular haemoglobin concentration
MCV	Mean corpuscular volume
MIBG	Meta-iodo-benzyl-guanine
MRI	Magnetic resonance imaging
MSU	Midstream urine
NBT	Nitroblue tetrazolium test
NCPAP	Nasal continuous positive airway pressure
NCS	Nerve conduction study
NH_4	Ammonia
NPA	Naso-pharyngeal aspirate
NS	Normal saline
O_2	Oxygen
OFC	Occipitofrontal circumference
PA	Pulmonary artery
Pb	Lead
PCO_2	Carbon dioxide tension
PCV	Packed cell volume
PDA	Patent ductus arteriosus
PEEP	Peak end-expiratory pressure
PEFR	Peak expiratory flow rate
pH	Logarithmic hydrogen ion concentration
PHA	Phytohaemoagglutinin
PHH	Post-haemorrhagic hydrocephalus
Plt	Platelets
PO_2	Oxygen tension
PO_4	Phosphate

PT	Prothrombin time
PTT	Partial thromboplastin time
RA	Right atrium
RAST	Radioallergosorbent test
RBBB	Right bundle branch block
Ret	Reticulocytes
RNA	Ribonucleic acid
RR	Respiratory rate
RV	Right ventricle
Sat	Saturation
SVC	Superior vena cava
SVT	Supraventricular tachycardia
SXR	Skull X-ray
T_4	Thyroxine
TAPVD	Total anomalous pulmonary venous drainage
TGA	Transposition of great arteries
TSH	Thyroid stimulating hormone
TT	Thrombin time
TV	Tidal volume
U	Urea
UAC	Umbilical artery catheter
U&E	Urea and electrolytes
US	Ultrasound
UTI	Urinary tract infection
UVC	Umbilical venous catheter
VC	Vital capacity
VEP	Visual evoked potential
VMA	Vanillylmandelic acid
VSD	Ventricular septal defect
VUR	Vesico-ureteric reflux
WCC	White cell count (N—neutrophils,L—lymphocytes, E—eosinophils, M—monocytes)

Case 1

35-week-old preterm infant. Born at 25 weeks' gestation, ventilated from day 1 to day 27 and on NCPAP of 3.9 cm water pressure in 40–55% O_2 until day 66. Now on nasal cannula with 0.1 l/min O_2.

Latest results are as follows:

Capillary blood gas

PO_2	4.03 kPa
PCO_2	9.12 kPa
pH	7.33
HCO_3	22 kPa
Be	3.4
Alk.ph	900 IU/l
ALT	13 IU/l
Albumin	31 g/l
Urea	2.5 mmol/l
Creatinine	28 µmol/l
Bilirubin	22 µmol/l
Na	133 mmol/l
K	4.5 mmol/l
Ca	2.14 mmol/l
PO_4	1.19 mmol/l
Mg	0.93 mmol/l

1. What does the capillary blood gas show?
2. What is the most likely diagnosis?
3. What other investigations would you perform?

Case 2

Cardiac catheterization was performed in a 6-year-old girl and a heart murmur was noticed.

	Pressure (mmHg)	Saturation %
SVC	5	70
RA	5	73
RV	60/5	86
PA	60/20	85
LA	11	93
LV	103/60	91
AO	103/60	92

1. What is the diagnosis?
2. Should the child be excluded from exercise at school?
3. How should this child be followed up?

Case 3

An 8-month-old girl presented with history of lethargy, cough and fever for 24 hours. She visited her GP and was diagnosed as having an URTI. Oral amoxycillin was commenced for 5 days. There was no improvement in her condition. She became more lethargic and unwell. At this point her GP referred her to hospital for further opinion. She had also developed bruises.

On examination pallor, cervical lymphadenopathy and hepatosplenomegaly were found.

Hb	5.9 g/dl
WCC	$16.4 \times 10^9/l$ (90% blasts)
Plt	$66 \times 109/l$
INR	0.94
PTT	43.5 (35–44 s)

1. What is the diagnosis?
2. What investigations are required to confirm the diagnosis?
3. What is the immediate management?

Case 4

An 11-year-old girl presented with a history of difficulty in breathing over a period of 25 days. RR 35, SaO_2 90–92 in air, BP 110/70, temperature 37.2°C and no lymphadenopathy. Bronchodilators were prescribed without benefit. Chest movement and air entry on the left side were reduced with dull percussion notes.

Hb	12.2 g/dl
WCC	$20.2 \times 10^9/l$ (N 43%, L 37%, E 17%, M 2.7%)
Plt	$390 \times 10^9/l$

Pleural aspirate performed for diagnostic and treatment purposes:

Protein	46 mmol/l
Lymphocytes	++++
Organisms	None
Cytology	Abnormal lymphocytes
AAFB	Negative
Culture	Negative

1. List the three most likely differential diagnoses.
2. Which two investigations would you perform next?

Case 5

A 6-year-old boy presents with a 4-week history of early morning headache and vomiting. Both parents are healthy and they own a horse-riding school. The boy shows normal development and good performance at school. He is withdrawn and does not initiate conversation by himself. He is described by his mother as being clumsy in the last 4 weeks.

Pulse	60/min
RR	20/min
BP	130/70 mmHg
Hb	13.3 g/dl
WCC	13.7×10^9/l (N 8.3)
Plt	534×10^9/l
Na	140 mmol/l
K	3.9 mmol/l
U	6.5 mmol/l
Cr	25 µmol/l

1. What is the most likely diagnosis?
2. List three possible causes.
3. State one investigation as your first choice.

Case 6

These are the results following an ITT, TRH, and LHRH in a short 12-year-old boy.

			Time/min			
	0	20	30	60	90	120
Glucose (mmol/l)	5.2	1.8	5.9	7.4	8.6	8.8
Cortisol (nmol/l)	507	—	1058	1378	1033	778
GH (mU/l)	16	8.2	7.1	6.1	4.0	13
TSH (mU/l)	2.0	13	—	8.4	—	—
FSH (u/l)	0.6	—	2.6	3.6	—	—
LH (u/l)	1	—	5.6	4.8	—	—

1. What is the diagnosis?
2. Which one further investigation is indicated?
3. Suggest two underlying causes.

Case 7

An 11-year-old girl presents with history of bloody diarrhoea, intermittent abdominal pain and wrist pain for the last three days. Weight and height are on the 75th and 50th centiles respectively. The rest of the examination is normal.

Hb	9.5 g/dl
WCC	$7.9 \times 10^9/l$
Plt	$656 \times 10^9/l$
ESR	58 mm/h
Serum iron	4.1 (4–10)

Red cell folate/vitamin B_{12} were normal

1.   What is the most likely diagnosis?
2.   Name one test to support your clinical diagnosis.
3.   What organ needs to be monitored regularly?

Case 8

These are the lung functions of a child having difficulty in breathing:

	Predicted	Measured	%
FVC (l)	2.41	1.91	79
FEV_1 (l)	2.19	1.76	81
FEV_1/FVC (%)	91	92	2
PEF (l/min)	314	275	88
FEF% (l/s)	1.29	1.14	89

1.   What disease does the child suffer from?
2.   What is the most likely cause?

Case 9

A 2-month-old infant presented with failure to thrive (FTT) and neonatal hypoglycaemia. Hepatosplenomegaly was noted on examination.

Hb	12.5 g/dl
WCC	$5.6 \times 10^9/l$
Plt	$56 \times 10^9/l$
Triglyceride	14.5 mmol/l (0.6–1.7 mmol/l)
Cholesterol	8.4 mmol/l (3.1–6.8 mmol/l)
Glucose	3.3 mmol/l
Urine uric acid	3.6 mmol/l (< 2 mmol/l)

1.   What is the most likely diagnosis?
2.   What are the diagnostic tests?
3.   What is the prognosis?

Case 10

A 12-year-old boy with Down's syndrome presented to A & E with history of being lethargic and sleepy and having a temperature of 38.3°C. Following admission he became more lethargic and developed generalised seizures.

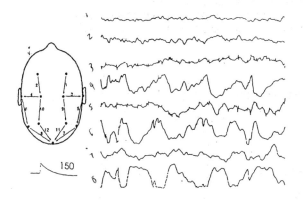

1. Describe the EEG abnormalities.
2. What is the most likely diagnosis?
3. Name one investigation to support your diagnosis.

ANSWERS 1–10

Case 1

1. Compensated respiratory acidosis
2. Bronchopulmonary dysplasia and metabolic bone disease
3. Wrist X-ray, echocardiography, ECG, and eye examination

Respiratory acidosis

Pathophysiology
Respiratory acidosis results from inadequate pulmonary excretion of carbon dioxide (CO_2) in the presence of normal production of CO_2. CO_2 is a major component of the principal buffer system of extracellular fluid. Any rise in CO_2 should be buffered by non-bicarbonate buffers, e.g. protein, phosphate, haemoglobin, and lactate within the cell and protein in the extracellular fluid.

An increase in CO_2 and acidosis will stimulate the kidneys to increase hydrogen ion excretion as well as ammonium and titratable acid. This will lead to more bicarbonate production as well as absorption. Then the level of bicarbonate will increase as a result of these physiological changes. The increase in plasma bicarbonate level compensates for the primary increase of CO_2 so the pH returns towards normal and respiratory acidosis is compensated by a normal renal mechanism.

Respiratory acidosis can be due to neuromuscular disorders, airway obstruction, vascular disease, pulmonary oedema and prematurity.

Chronic lung disease of prematurity (CLDP) is mainly obstructive and leads to chronic respiratory acidosis which can be compensated by normal renal function through the buffering mechanism.

CLDP is defined as O_2 dependence and signs of respiratory distress at a post-conception age of 36 weeks (Shennan et al 1988).

Different features of acid–base balance:

	pH	PCO_2	PO_2	HCO_3
Metabolic acidosis	Low	Normal	Low	Low
Respiratory acidosis	Low or normal	High	Low	High or normal
Metabolic alkalosis	High	High or normal	Low or normal	High
Respiratory alkalosis	High	Low	Low or normal	Low

Case 2

1. Ventricular septal defect (VSD) with increased pulmonary pressure
2. Yes
3. Echocardiography every 6 months with ECG and/or chest X-ray; growth assessment

Ventricular septal defect (VSD)

The results of cardiac catheterisation show that the blood in the right ventricle is higher in oxygen content than that in the right atrium. The oxygen content of blood in the pulmonary artery is slightly higher. If the VSD is large then the pulmonary blood flow is high with equal systemic and pulmonary pressures.

Normal values for cardiac catheterisation:

	RA	LA	RV	LV	PA	Aorta
SaO_2	65%	99%	65%	98%	65%	97%
Pressure	4 mmHg	6 mmHg	25/4 mmHg	75/6 mmHg	25/15 mmHg	75/7 mmHg

About 40–50% of small VSDs close spontaneously before the first birthday. Spontaneous closure is less common in moderate and large defects even if the VSD becomes smaller as the child grows up. A small percentage of patients (2%) are at risk of developing endocarditis. Prophylactic antibiotics are necessary in patients who need dental surgery, tonsillectomy, adenoidectomy, or instrumentation of the genito-urinary and gastrointestinal system. This risk is independent of the size of the VSD.

There is no restriction on physical activity of children with VSD if there is no evidence of raised pulmonary hypertension. They should be allowed to participate in sport activity according to their ability. A few patients develop elevated pulmonary arterial pressure as a result of an increase in pulmonary blood flow if the repair is not performed early in large VSDs.

Management
Medical management in patients with large VSDs is by treating chest infection, adequate nutrition with regular follow-up, and diuretics if required. If this fails, then surgery should be performed early rather than late. The prognosis is excellent following surgery.

Case 3

1. Acute lymphoblastic leukaemia (ALL)
2. Bone marrow aspiration (BMA) and trephine for cytology and cell markers
3. • Blood transfusion
   • Platelet transfusion
   • Hyperhydration with 4% dextrose, 0.18% NS
   • Allopurinol, antibiotics

Prognostic features for ALL

Good prognosis	Poor prognosis
> 1 and < 10 years old	< 1 and > 10 years old
Girls	Boys
WCC < 20 × 10^9/l	> 40 × 10^9/l
C-ALL	B-ALL
	Positive Philadelphia chromosome

The incidence of ALL is 70–75% of all child leukaemias. The peak incidence of ALL is usually at the age of 4 years. Patients with ALL are subclassified according to the morphological and immunological features of blast cells as well as clinical presentation.

The cytological markers are L_1, L_2, and L_3 cells. The cell membrane markers according to the monoclonal antibodies on the blast cells, e.g. CD5, CD7, indicate T-cell type.

The translocation is a valuable marker for prognosis.

Remission is achieved by:

a. induction chemotherapy course to clear bone marrow of blast cells
b. prophylactic CNS therapy
c. continuation therapy for 2–3 years.

Case 4

1. Lymphomas
   Pulmonary tuberculosis
   Systemic lupus erythematosus
2. Lymph node biopsy
   Chest CT scan

Lymphomas

Lymphomas rarely occur before the age of 5 years and are more frequent in boys. The incidence peaks at the age of 15–35 years and again over the age of 50 years.

The histological classification is as follows:

a. Lymphocytosis, with a good prognosis, occurs in 20% of total Hodgkin's disease (HD).
b. Nodular sclerosis is the commonest form and has a good prognosis.
c. The mixed type, which includes lymphocytes, plasma cells and Reed–Sternberg cells, is the second commonest type.
d. Lymphocyte depletion has a poor prognosis and occurs in 10% of total HD.

Four stages of the disease have been defined:

Each stage can be divided into A (without fever or weight loss at presentation) or B (with fever and weight loss).

CT scanning of the chest and abdomen is used for staging. If laboratory staging has been used then splenectomy is performed with lymph node biopsy above and below the diaphragm. The cure rate is 90%. Both chemotherapy and radiotherapy are effective modes of treatment.

- Stages I & II—curable with chemotherapy
- Stage III—75% cure rate with radiotherapy and chemotherapy
- Stage IV—50% cure rate following intensive chemotherapy.

1–2% of patients with splenectomy are in danger of developing fatal sepsis with *Strep. pneumoniae* and *H. influenzae*. The pneumococcal vaccine and prophylactic antibiotics (penicillin) should be given to these patients. Less than 5% of patients may develop secondary 'leukaemic' changes.

Case 5

1. Space occupying lesion (tumour)
2. Intracranial tumour
   Brain abscess
   Benign intracranial hypertension
3. MRI with gadolinium

Raised intracranial pressure
The history of vomiting, anorexia and headache over the preceding 4 weeks with changes in personality and bilateral papilloedema indicate an increase in intracranial pressure. The diagnostic possibilities include a space occupying lesion (tumour), brain abscess, intracranial bleed or benign intracranial hypertension.

A brain tumour is the most likely cause of raised intracranial pressure in this case. Infratentorial tumours are more common than supratentorial tumours.

Supratentorial tumours
These occur more commonly in the under 2-year age group and again in adolescents. About 40% are of glial origin (astrocytoma, ependymoma and oligodendroglioma). Oligodendroglioma occurs exclusively in the cerebral hemispheres and is rare during childhood. This tumour grows slowly and usually calcifies. Astrocytoma and ependymoma may be found in either a supratentorial or infratentorial position.

Infratentorial tumours
Medulloblastoma is common in children < 7 years of age and is one of the primitive neuroectodermal tumours (PNET) with the capacity to differential into neuronal and glial tissue. Most arise from the vermis or fourth ventricle with or without extension to the cerebellar hemispheres. About 90% present in the first decade. The tumour grows rapidly and the time between the onset of symptoms and medical examination is generally brief: 2 weeks in 25% and less than a month in 50%. Vomiting is the initial presentation in 60%. The high risk group with poor prognosis comprises those where there is any evidence of tumour dissemination, tumours invading two structures or filling the fourth ventricle and extending to the third ventricle or cervical spine. Medulloblastomas are more radio-sensitive than gliomas. When the combination of surgery, radiotherapy and chemotherapy is used in the treatment of medulloblastoma, the 5-year survival rate is 50–70%.

Case 6

1. Partial growth hormone insufficiency
2. CT scan with contrast or MRI of the brain
3. Pituitary tumour, septo-optic dysplasia

Growth hormone (GH) insufficiency
A normal growth hormone response is accepted as > 15–20 mU/l depending on the assay. A partial response with levels < 7 mU/l is a GH deficiency.

Other causes of short stature should be excluded prior to performing a GH provocation test. These include chronic illness, chronic renal failure and renal tubular acidosis. Additional endocrine causes such as hypothyroidism should be excluded:

Congenital: Idiopathic growth hormone releasing hormone deficiency, pituitary hypoplasia, mid-facial defect and pituitary aplasia, GH gene deletion, acquired hypothalamic or pituitary tumours, cranial irradiation, head injuries, infection (meningitis encephalitis), hypothyroidism.

Transient: Low sex hormone concentration, psycho-social deprivation (C. Brook).

In growth hormone deficiency or insufficiency, the growth velocity is poor and the height less than 2SD of the mean. The bone age is delayed and the clinical appearance may be characterised by increased skin fold thickening, infantile 'doll-like facies' and micropenis.

The use of growth hormone in these children will restore a normal growth velocity after a period of catch-up growth. If the patient does not respond to the treatment, either the compliance is poor or the diagnosis may be wrong.

IGF-1 levels can be helpful in the diagnosis and to assess compliance. When testing a child for growth hormone deficiency in the prepubertal years with no signs of puberty, the child should be primed with sex steroids 2 days before the test (testosterone 100 mg for boys and ethinyl oestradiol 30 mg for girls).

Causes of childhood short stature

Familial	Genetic short stature (parents' height and sibling if possible) Constitutional delay
Nutritional	Intrauterine growth retardation (neonatal and infant period growth charts)
Chronic disease	GIT (inflammatory bowel disease, coeliac disease) Cardiac (cyanotic and chronic heart failure) Lung (cystic fibrosis, uncontrolled asthma) Renal (chronic renal failure, RTA) Bone and cartilage (JCA, SLE, dysplasia) Hepatic (chronic hepatitis) Blood (thalassaemia, sickle cell anaemia) Brain (post irradiation, tumours)
Hormonal	Growth hormone deficiency Hypothyroidism Turner's syndrome Sexual precocity Steroids
Emotional deprivation	Family and social history

Case 7

1. Inflammatory bowel disease
2. Endoscopy of upper and lower GIT with biopsy
3. Eyes

Inflammatory bowel disease

A peptic ulcer can present with high abdominal pain and faecal occult blood. However the joint pain and skin lesions suggest a systemic cause for the abdominal pain. Septic or juvenile chronic arthritis (JCA) rarely presents with abdominal pain, but in Still's disease it may be due to splenomegaly. The joints are red, hot, oedematous and tender in septic arthritis with effusion, a high ESR, CRP and polymorphonuclear leukocytosis.

The history of bloody diarrhoea, frequent abdominal pain and joint pains with a high ESR are all features of CIBD (Crohn's disease and ulcerative colitis).

Algorithm for the diagnosis of chronic diarrhoea

Stool culture and reducing substances, immunoglobulins RAST test	Infection, tropical sprue, protein intolerance, disaccharidase deficiency

↓ *negative*

Abdominal ultrasound and X-ray	Chronic constipation, toddler's diarrhoea

↓ *negative*

Sweat test, IRT, DNA linkage study (Δ508) Pancreatic enzyme deficiency	Cystic fibrosis

↓ *negative*

Low platelets, neutropenia, skeletal abnormalities Pancreatic enzyme deficiency	Schwachman's syndrome

↓ *negative*

Conjugated hyperbilirubinaemia Abnormal LFT and clotting, abdominal ultrasound	Biliary atresia

↓ *negative*

Small and large intestine biopsy, immunoglobulin levels	Crohn's, coeliac disease, immune deficiency, ulcerative colitis

Case 8

1. Restrictive lung disease
2. Neuromuscular disorders
   Fibrosing alveolitis

Lung function

	Obstructive	Restrictive
FVC	Low	Low
VC	Low	Low
FEV_1	Low	Low (proportion to FVC)
FEV_1/FVC	Low	Normal or high
$FEF_{25-75\%}$	Low	Low

Restrictive lung diseases
The common *causes* are cystic fibrosis, pulmonary infection, pulmonary oedema, fibrosing alveolitis, emphysema and neuromuscular disorders.

Obstructive lung diseases
The common *causes* are bronchiolitis, asthma, bronchiectasis and cystic fibrosis.

Case 9

1. Glycogen storage disease type IB (GSD type IB)
2. White cell enzyme
   Liver biopsy
3. Good

Glycogen storage diseases
The glycogen storage diseases are a group of autosomal recessive inherited disorders with multisystemic effects.

Several types of GSD have been described: generalised type IV (Pompe's disease), brain (GSD VIII), hepatic (GSD I, III, VI, IX), and muscle (GSD V, McArdle's disease).

Glycogen storage disease type IB (GSD type IB)

Clinical features
GSD type IB is similar to the common GSD type A with repeated clinical and laboratory findings except that GSD type IB is associated with neutropenia, thrombocytopenia and chronic inflammatory bowel disease. The activity of glucose-6-phosphatase is normal on liver biopsy. There is a transport defect of glucose-6-phosphatase at the microsomal membrane. The liver is enlarged, with glycogen

deposition in the kidney and normal mental development. Patients have a tendency to develop recurrent hypoglycaemia, lactic acidosis, hyperlipidaemia, hyperuricaemia, gout, bleeding and repeated infections.

Investigations
There is no rise in glucose level following a subcutaneous injection of ephedrine or intravenous glucagon, but lactic acidosis and hypoglycaemia can be present in other diseases when this test is performed, e.g. fructose-1-6-diphosphatase deficiency, pyruvate decarboxylase deficiency, and carnitine deficiency.

Treatment
The key to treating GSD type IB, A, or C is to ensure normoglycaemia throughout the 24-hour period. If this can be done then the secondary metabolic upsets—acidosis, high uric acid and cholesterol—will settle spontaneously with normal growth and development. In GSD type 1 A, B or C in particular, nocturnal intragastric feeding of glucose polymerase may be required as well as hourly drinks of glucose polymerase. This regime may cause increased sensitivity to hypoglycaemia, obesity and enuresis.

Case 10

1. Left temporal periodic slow waves
2. Herpes simplex encephalitis
3. Cranial computerized tomography

There are pathological changes in the brain consistent with haemorrhage, necrosis, and oedema with inflammatory cell infiltration.

EEG shows typical periodic complexes over the temporal lobe region with focal discharges.

CT scan of the head will show areas of low attenuation coincident with the changes on EEG most of the time. The CSF may show a rise in red cells or evidence of viral meningitis. The polymerase chain reaction test will be diagnostic but it will take 5–7 days to get the results back.

Acyclovir (30 mg/kg/day) is the current recommendation and shows good results. The results of treatment depend on the stage at which the treatment is started. Mortality is 15% in patients presenting with lethargy at the time of starting treatment, and 40% in comatose patients. All patients need to be treated in an intensive care unit; control of fits and fluid balance are important in the management of patients with HSV encephalitis. The prognosis for untreated cases is very poor with 70–80% mortality in the first 30 days post infection and up to 90% 4–6 weeks post infection.

Possibilities to consider in the differential diagnosis of acute encephalitis

Intracranial infection

Bacterial, tuberculous meningitis, brain abscess, cerebral oedema	Lumbar puncture, CT or MRI scan Mantoux test, BCG scar

↓

Metabolic disorders

Fluid, electrolytes and acid-based disorders, amino acid and organic acid disorders, urea cycle disorders, lactic acidosis	Electrolytes, blood gas, glucose, lactate, ammonia Amino acids Urine organic acids and amino acids

↓

Hypoxic-ischaemic injuries

Cardiorespiratory arrest, hypoxic-ischaemic encephalopathy, near-miss SIDS, shock	MRI or CT CXR, NPA, electrolytes, blood gas, glucose, ammonia, lactate EEG

↓

Vascular disease

Vascular malformation, embolic and vascular disease, venous thrombosis	MRI, diffuse weight MRI PT, PTT, TT, platelet function, Factor S, C, Laden MRA, venogram, arteriograph

↓

Seizure disorders

Status epilepticus, hemiconvulsions–hemiplegia syndrome, non convulsive status epilepticus	EEG, video telemetry, MRI scan

↓

Para-infectious encephalopathies

Reye's syndrome, haemorrhagic shock, haemorrhagic encephalopathy, toxic shock syndrome	Ammonia, blood gas, PT, PTT, TT, FBC, U&Es, EEG, CT or MRI Serum virology and blood culture

↓

Toxic injuries

Endogenous toxins (diabetes, uraemia, liver failure) Exogenous toxins (drugs and household agents)	Urea and electrolytes, plasma glucose, ammonia, LFT Urine toxicology

↓

Increased intracranial pressure

Increased intracranial pressure (tumours, haematomas, acute hydrocephalus, lead poisoning)	MRI or CT scan, lead plasma level, FBC

BMA Library

BMA House, Tavistock Square, London WC1H 9JP

British Medical Association
BMA House
Tavistock Square
London
WC1H 9JP

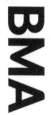

BMA

Case 11

This is the ECG of a 2-year-old girl with a history of vomiting and fast heart rate.

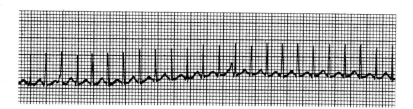

1. What two abnormalities show up on the ECG?
2. What is the most likely diagnosis?
3. Name three possible therapeutic procedures.

Case 12

A term baby boy was born vaginally at 2 am. One hour later the paediatrician was called to see the baby because of irritability and difficulty in breathing. The pregnancy had been normal and membrane rupture occurred 90 minutes before delivery. The baby had had no feed since birth. On examination he was grunting with marked subcostal and intercostal recession. Air entry was reduced on the left side of the chest.

1. List three possible diagnoses.
2. What one bedside investigation would you do immediately?
3. What subsequent investigations would you perform?

Case 13

A 2-year-old boy presents with diarrhoea followed by a period of constipation. There is a history of frequent ear and throat infections.

Hb	12.2 g/dl
WCC	7.1 × 10⁹/l (N 45%, L 37%)
Plt	320 × 10⁹/l
CD3	66%
CD4	42%
CD8	24%
CD19 (B-cells)	22%
CD3 + CD56	< 5%
IgG, IgA, IgE	Normal

Jejunal and colonic biopsies were normal. Stool culture was negative for bacteria and viruses, and there was no evidence of Giardia or protozoan infection.

1. Name one further investigation.
2. How would you treat this patient?

Case 14

A 4-year-old girl presented with bone pain.

Urine (24-hour collection)

VMA	71 mg/24 h	(normal < 10)
HVA	216 mg/24 h	(normal < 30)
Dopamine	1950	(normal 2700)
Hb	7 g/dl	
WCC	$6.8 \times 10^9/l$	
Plt	$205 \times 10^9/l$	

1. What is the most likely diagnosis?
2. Which three further investigations are indicated?

Case 15

A baby born at 27 weeks' gestation was ventilated from the age of 3 minutes and Curosurf given for moderate HMD. On day 5 the ventilator settings were as follows: rate 65/min, Ti 0.45 s, PIP/PEEP 20/3, FiO_2 60%.

UAC blood gas

pH	7.30
PCO_2	6.16 kPa
PO_2	5.6 kPa
Be	−5.1
MAP	36 mmHg without inotropic support

Two hours later the O_2 requirement increased and the baby became bradycardic.

1. Describe your immediate management.

An arterial blood gas was taken at this time and showed the following:

pH	7.25
PCO_2	6.80 kPa
PO_2	3.06 kPa
Be	−9.6

2. What does the abnormality in the blood gas show?
3. How would you change the ventilator setting to correct the abnormality?

Case 16

The following are the results of cardiac catheterisation in a 3-day-old boy with congenital heart disease.

O_2 saturation %		Pressure (mmHg)	
PA	83	PA	24
PV	97	LA	10
LA	95	LV	104/10
LV	89		
AO	82	AO	79

1. What is the diagnosis?
2. What is the current treatment?

Case 17

A 3-week-old baby was admitted with history of drowsiness, lethargy and hypothermia.

Hb	16.5
WCC	$3.3 \times 10^9/l$ (N 300)
Plt	$11 \times 10^9/l$
U	6.1 mmol/l
Cr	109 µmol/l
K	4.3 mmol
Na	136 mmol/l
Glucose	5.3 mmol/l
pH	7.32
PO_2	7.9 kPa
PCO_2	4.6 kPa
HCO_3	19 kPa
Be	−6
Plasma lactate	4.1 mmol/l

1. What are the possible diagnoses?
2. Would you carry out a lumbar puncture, and, if so, why?
3. Name three first line management measures.

Case 18

A 5-week-old boy presented with a history of recurrent seizures. Echocardiography showed cardiomyopathy. Urine gas chromatography and mass spectroscopy showed raised propionyl glycine and 3-hydroxy propionate. There was a slight rise in lactate and pyruvate. His ammonia level was high and required peritoneal dialysis.

1. What is the diagnosis?
2. What is the regimen for feeding?
3. Of what other risk factors should you warn the parents?

Case 19

A 9-year-old albino boy has a history of increasing puffiness on his face and body for the last 5 days. There is a history of 3 days of upper respiratory tract infection. The urine is dark in colour with hyaline cast.

Na	131 mmol/l
K	4.6 mmol/l
U	12 mmol/l
Cr	110 μmol/l
BP	128/85 on several occasions

Passed 400 ml urine in last 24 hours

1. What is the diagnosis?
2. What is the underlying cause?

Case 20

This is the family tree of a family with blood disorders.

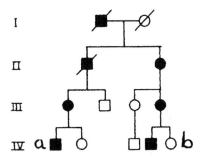

1. What is the inheritance?
2. What is the sibling risk of getting the same condition?
   a.
   b.
3. Give two examples of blood diseases inherited in the same way.

ANSWERS 11–20

Case 11

1. Heart rate 300/min. No P wave and P wave buried in the T wave.
2. Supraventricular tachycardia
3. Carotid sinus massage
   Submerge face in cold water or put an ice bag on the face
   IV adenosine

Management of SVT
Heart rate > 240/min, narrow QRS complex

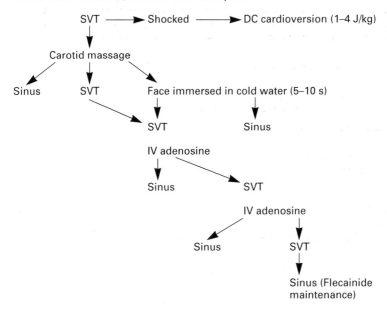

Adenosine blocks conduction through the AV node. It is not contraindicated in asthmatic patients and should be avoided in patients with AV block. Adenosine will not convert SVT arising from atrial abnormalities to sinus rhythm and it may increase block in these circumstances. Adenosine is not a preventive agent.

Pathophysiology of SVT
There is an abnormally fast heart rate arising from or caused by an abnormality in a site above the ventricles. The common cause of SVT is re-entry phenomena through the accessory pathway, as in AV re-entry tachycardia, or within the AV node. Atrioventricular re-entry tachycardia is common in early childhood and fetal life and due to an accessory pathway (Wolff–Parkinson–White syndrome). ECG is diagnostic during the episode. Tachycardia with narrow complexes is usually SVT. P waves are mostly detectable halfway between each QRS complex in infantile SVT. In other forms, P waves may be not present or be very close to the QRS complex or buried in the T wave. If broad complexes are present then ventricular tachycardia should be first on the list, except if the patient is known to have bundle branch block while in sinus rhythm. The SVT can be classified according to the origin of the rhythm: sinus node, atrial muscle, or AV junction. The differential diagnosis from atrial flutter, atrial fibrillation, atrial tachycardia and sinus tachycardia can be ascertained by ECG.

Case 12

1. Sepsis
    Pneumothorax
    Diaphragmatic hernia
2. Chest illumination
3. Chest X-ray
    Septic screen

Pneumothorax in the term newborn infant

Actions to be taken while the baby is being ventilated if oxygen requirement is increased:

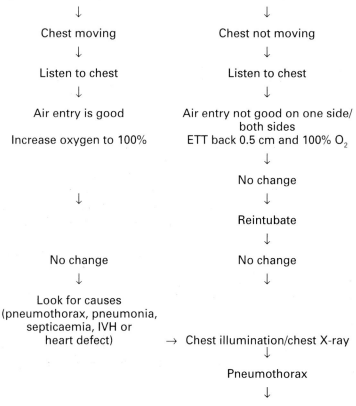

Pneumothorax is estimated to occur in up to 1–2% of term infants. The commonest cause is alveolar rupture due to overinflation. It can occur spontaneously. Symptomatic pneumothorax is characterised by respiratory distress (increase in RR, apnoea, tachypnoea and cyanosis with grunting). Sudden deterioration is uncommon. Gradual deterioration in respiratory function is the most commonly observed scenario in term infants. Chest movement may be asymmetric with decreased air entry on the affected side and mediastinal shift to the opposite side if the pneumothorax is unilateral. Bilateral pneumothoraces are difficult to diagnose clinically. Transillumination of the chest wall and CXR are vital diagnostic tools.

Administration of 100% oxygen can accelerate the re-absorption of free pleural air into the blood by reducing the nitrogen tension in blood. This will produce a nitrogen gradient pressure from the trapped air into the blood. The risk of oxygen toxicity should be borne in mind and weighed up against the benefit of treating the pneumothorax by giving 100% oxygen.

Case 13

1. Assessment of IgG subclass deficiency
2. Treat infection (may need longer course of antibiotics)
   Consider Sandoglobulin infusion on a monthly basis

IgG subclasses deficiency
The biopsies are normal, excluding inflammatory bowel disease, coeliac disease and infective causes. The stools are normal, excluding any infestation cause. The B and T cell function are normal. The history of repeated ear infection and sore throat would indicate an immunological problem. IgG subclasses should be assessed.

The cluster of differentiation (CD) represents the T and B cells of the immune system. CD2, 3, 4, 8 and 25 represent T cells, and CD 19 and 21 represent B cells.

IgG subclass deficiency can present with repeated ear infection. There are four subtypes—IgG1–4. The deficiency may be partial or complete. It may also be associated with IgA deficiency. IgG1–3 deficiency increases susceptibility to respiratory infection. IgG1 deficiency is the most severe and may lead to chronic progressive lung disease. IgG2 deficiency responds to polysaccharide antigen and is commonly associated with IgA and/or IgG4 deficiency. IgG4 deficiency alone has no significance. The total IgG level is usually low in IgG1 deficiency, but within normal levels in other IgG subclass deficiencies.

Case 14

1. Neuroblastoma
2. Abdominal and chest CT scan
   Bone marrow biopsy
   Meta-iodo-benzyl-guanidine (MIBG) scan

Neuroblastoma
Bony tenderness with raised dopamine metabolites VMA and HVA in the urine suggests a neural crest lesion; the commonest lesion in childhood is a neuroblastoma. Phaeochromocytoma is rare.

Clinical features
Neuroblastoma usually presents as an abdominal mass. In 10% of patients, it can present with dancing eye syndrome (opsoclonus–myoclonus syndrome). This myoclonic encephalopathy (opsoclonus–myoclonus syndrome) is characterised by chaotic eye movements, myoclonic ataxia and encephalopathy; it may be idiopathic or occur as the result of an occult neuroblastoma. MRI of the chest and abdomen to diagnose occult neuroblastoma is indicated.

ACTH or oral corticosteroids provide partial or complete relief of symptoms in 80% of patients, including patients with neuroblastoma.

Investigations
Homovanillic acid (HVA) and vanillylmandelic acid (VMA) levels in urine, and dopa, dopamine, norepinephrine and normetanephrine levels in serum are high in 90% of children with neuroblastoma. These can be assayed by mass spectrography and gas chromatography; the tests are sensitive, even if the urine or serum samples are small in quantity. A 24-hour urine collection is required to prove the diagnosis, even when mass spectrography and chromatography tests are used. The secretion of catecholamine metabolites is much higher in children with phaeochromocytoma than in those with neuroblastoma. Meta-iodo-benzyl-guanidine (MIBG) can be taken up by catecholamine producing tumours and used to locate the primary tumour and metastatic lesions. Biopsy of the lesion and bone marrow trephine biopsy are the definitive diagnostic tests.

Case 15

1.   Check ETT, CXR, chest illumination
2.   Metabolic acidosis
3.   Increase PEEP and RR

Sudden deterioration in the previously stable condition of a premature baby should raise suspicion of a technical fault or an acute complication. The position of the endotracheal tube should be checked to ensure adequate air entry.

Transillumination of the chest is vital to exclude pneumothorax. A blood gas analysis and Hem-cue test are other tests which can be done quickly. Immediate manoeuvres to improve oxygenation should include an increase in inspiratory time and PEEP. A septic screen and U&E analysis should be performed. Chest X-ray should be ordered, and head ultrasound may be indicated as an intraventricular haemorrhage could be responsible for the sudden deterioration.

If the pH drops below 7.1, correction of metabolic acidosis using bicarbonate may be indicated but be aware of increase in CO_2 and Na. The acidosis should be half-corrected as an infusion. This can all be done with consultation with senior colleagues if needed.

Case 16

1.   Transposition of the great arteries (TGA with VSD)
2.   Switch operation with VSD closure

Assessment of a newborn or child with suspected congenital heart disease

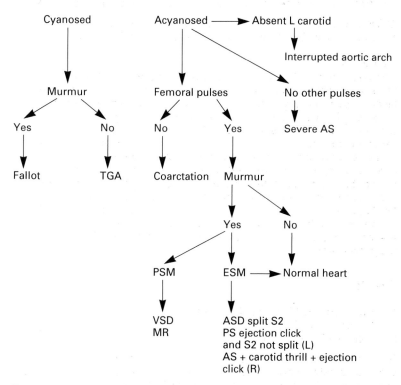

Key:
AS Aortic stenosis
ASD Atrial septal defect
ESM Ejection systolic murmur
(L) Left sternal edge
MR Mitral regurgitation
PS Pulmonary stenosis
PSM Pansystolic murmur
(R) Right sternal edge
TGA Transposition of great arteries
VSD Ventricular septal defect

Transposition of great vessels (TGA)
Saturation in the aorta is lower than that in the pulmonary artery, and is also lower than in the other chambers of the heart.

Management
- Keep the duct open by giving a prostaglandin infusion
- Correct metabolic acidosis
- Ventilation may be required, especially if the baby is transferred to another unit
- Give diuretics if in failure
- Give inotropic drugs if blood pressure is not maintained
- Atrial septostomy can be done later by an experienced cardiologist
- Total correction can be performed at any time, preferably early

Case 17

1. Sepsis
   Meningitis
2. No (platelets are low)
3. Intravenous fluid (40 ml/kg crystalloid; if more is needed, give colloid)

   IV broad-spectrum antibiotics
   Check clotting and correct if abnormal
   Check capillary or arterial gas

Septicaemia
It is difficult to distinguish between different illnesses in the neonatal period. Many of them result in non-specific symptoms such as fever, hypothermia, lethargy, poor feeding, drowsiness, seizures, crying and irritability, diarrhoea, vomiting, and tachycardia or bradycardia as well as apnoea. Infection should be ruled out by performing a full septic screen including a lumbar puncture. The septic screen should also include a full blood count with differential white cell counts, C-reactive protein, blood culture, chest X-ray, urine microscopy and culture. A blood glucose level should be checked in order to eliminate hypoglycaemia. The baby should be commenced on broad-spectrum antibiotics for 48 hours pending culture results.

When infection has been excluded and if the child is still not improving, or if there is a family history of metabolic diseases, arterial or capillary gas should also be assessed. A urea cycle defect (high level of ammonia) and an organic acidaemia (high plasma ketone, hypoglycaemia, high ammonia and profound metabolic acidosis) are first to present during the early neonatal period. CSF lactate is important in mitochondrial cytopathy if suspected. All these tests can be done as a baseline in the exclusion of metabolic disorders. Further detailed tests can be done in a specialised centre if a metabolic disorder is still the main diagnosis.

Case 18

1. Propionic acidaemia
2. Low protein diet
   Carnitine supplement
   Increased calorie intake
3. Sudden infant death syndrome (SIDS)

Organic acidaemias
This is a group of disorders inherited in an autosomal recessive fashion and presenting as severe neonatal illness. It is characterised by heavy ketonuria, which is unusual in the neonatal period, and marked metabolic acidosis with a large anion gap. There is a moderate rise in ammonia. There may be a history of a sibling having died from infection or sudden infant death syndrome.

Propionic acidaemia
This is one of the commonest organic acid disorders and is due to a deficiency of propionyl-CoA carboxylase. Pregnancy and birth are usually normal. The infant starts to deteriorate hours or days after birth with poor feeding, vomiting, hypotonia, lethargy and dehydration. The infant is acidotic and may progress to coma and death if prompt treatment is not introduced. The severe form occurs in 30% of affected infants, and the severity of symptoms varies within families. It is also associated with neutropenia and thrombocytopenia due to a toxic effect on the bone marrow which may mislead the clinician in the direction of another diagnosis, e.g. septicaemia.

Hypoglycaemia and slightly elevated serum ammonia levels are two further features of this condition. Hyperglycinaemia is common in these patients and can be found in other organic acid disorders (methylmalonic acidaemia, isovaleric acidaemia, β-ketothiolase deficiency). The diagnosis can be established by screening urine for organic acid, white cell enzyme assay, and skin biopsy for fibroblast culture.

Treatment
The emergency treatment includes peritoneal dialysis, a protein intake of 0.25 mg/kg/day, gut sterilisation, L-carnitine as the patients later become carnitine deficient due to excessive urinary organic aciduria, and reduction of ammonia level by dialysis or sodium benzoate. Some children may be left with a permanent neurological deficit. Long-term therapy is based on a low protein diet and avoidance of stressful conditions, e.g. infection, starvation or long surgical procedures.

Case 19

1. Acute nephritis
2. Post-streptococcal acute glomerulonephritis

Acute glomerulonephritis

Investigations

Urine:

- Haematuria, smoky-grey to reddish brown (Hb to acid haematin)
- Proteinuria trace up to 100 mg/dl
- Red blood cell cast in 80% of patients

Blood:

- Blood urea nitrogen (BUN) and creatinins raised in a significant number of patients
- ASO titres raised
- C3 low

Kidney ultrasound is normal. A throat or skin swab may be positive for A β-haemolytic streptococci.

Classifications of glomerulonephritis:

	C3	C4	Immune complex
Membranous GN	Normal	Normal	Variable
Membranous proliferative GN	Reduced	Reduced	Present
Focal segmental GN	Normal	Normal	Not present
IgA nephropathy	Normal	Normal	Present
SLE	Reduced	Reduced	Present
Henoch-Schönlein purpura	Normal	Normal	Variable
Diabetes mellitus	Normal	Normal	Normal
Polyarteritis nodosa	Normal	Normal	Not present
Acute post-streptococcal GN	Reduced	Normal	Present

Case 20

1. Autosomal dominant
2.
   a. 50%
   b. Nil
3. Spherocytosis
   Haemoglobin variants

Case 21

A 2-week-old infant presented with heart failure, which is under treatment with diuretics and digoxin. Echocardiography data showed:

	Pressure (mmHg)
LV	94/26 = systolic/diastolic—mean (60)
Descending aorta	67/43
Across AV	40
RV & RA	12
SaO_2 AO	100% in LV

1. What is the diagnosis?
2. What is the most immediate action to be taken?

Case 22

An ataxic 5-year-old boy was seen in the paediatric neurology clinic. Investigations include:

FBC + film	Normal
MRI	Normal
Amino acids and organic acids	Normal
Alpha-fetoprotein	80 mmol/l (10–30 mmol/l)
Plasma lactate	2.1 normal
CSF lactate	1.2 normal
Very long chain fatty acids	Normal
Nerve conduction study and EMG	Normal

1. What is the diagnosis?
2. List two other clinical signs which should be looked for.
3. List three other investigations.

Case 23

A 3-year-old girl presented with diarrhoea and vomiting for the last 5 days. She was pale and lethargic, and stools tested positive for blood.

Hb	8.8 g/dl
WCC	25.5×10^9/l (N 18.7, L 6.7)
Plt	55×10^9/l
U	21 mmol/l
Na	117 mmol/l
K	5.2 mmol/l
Cr	200 mmol/l
PT	16 s (12–14)
PTT	29.5 s (27–40)
TT	13 s (9–11)

1. What is the diagnosis?
2. What other three investigations can be done?
3. What is the underlying cause?

Case 24

A term infant girl was born with myotonic dystrophy and ventilated for 77 days. She was fed via a nasogastric tube. Before each feed, 15–25 ml of milk was aspirated from the stomach. During the ward round she self-extubated and was successfully reintubated with an ETT size 4.5 mm. Three hours later her oxygen requirement increased from 55% to 100% with frequent desaturation.

1. What would you do at this stage?
2. Give one cause for her sudden deterioration.

Case 25

A 5-month-old girl has an advanced bone age with height on the 90th centile.

Testosterone	1.1 nmol/l	(pre-pubertal below 8 nmol/l)
Androstenedione	6.1 nmol/l	(pre-pubertal below 1.0 nmol/l)
DHA-sulphate	1.4 µmol/l	(pre-pubertal below 0.5 µmol/l)
FSH	< 3.0 U/l	
LH	< 1.9 U/l	

1. What is the conclusion?
2. What is the most likely underlying cause?
3. What is the most important investigation?

Case 26

A 3-year-old boy with history of dark urine has been unable to walk for the last 12 hours. His demeanour is unhappy.

Hb	11.7 g/dl
WCC	11.9×10^9/l (N 6.7, L 4.9)
Plt	156×10^9/l
PT	11 s (12–14)
PTT	30 s (27–38)
TT	8 min (9–11)
Fib	3.6 (3.2–4.3)
Na	136 mmol/l
K	4.1 mmol/l
U	5.6 mmol/l
Cr	37 µmol/l
Alb	28 g/l
Alk.ph	78 IU/l

ALT   8860 IU/l
Blood film   Normal
AST   1330 IU/l
CK   80

1. Why is he unable to walk?
2. What are the next three investigations you would perform?
3. List three possible underlying causes.

Case 27

This is an EEG of a 10-year-old boy with history of clumsiness and progressive poor performance at school. Previous medical history of measles and chicken pox.

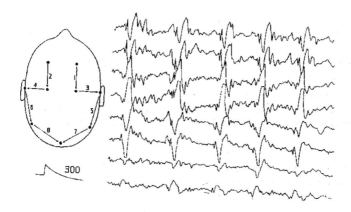

1. What abnormalities are on the EEG?
2. What is the diagnosis?
3. What is the prognosis and how could it be avoided?

Case 28

The followings results are for a 10-year-old patient with a history of jaundice and abdominal distension. On examination there was hepatosplenomegaly with firm consistency.

Na   136
K   3.4
Ca   2.27
PO_4 0.91
Hb   11.6 g/dl
WCC 2.80×10^9/l normal differential
Plt 69×10^9/l
PT   17 (16)

PTT	43 (33)
Alk.ph	786 IU/l
Protein	69 g/l
Alb	34 g/l
ALT	510 IU/l
AST	786 IU/l
Copper	13 µmol/l (11–15)
HBsAg	Negative
HBab	Negative
IgA	5.6 g/l (0.7–3)
IgG	10.7 g/l (6.5–16)
IgM	1.05 g/l (0.7–2.8)
γ-glutamyl transpeptidase	124 IU/l
ESR	22 mm/h
α_1-antitrypsin	43 µmol/l (20–40)

There was no evidence of storage diseases.

1. What is the most likely diagnosis?
2. How would you confirm it?

Case 29

A 2-month-old infant has an URTI which is not responding to treatment by amoxycillin. He is also having apnoeic episodes.

Hb	11.9 g/dl
WCC	36×10^9/l (N 31%, L 65%, M 2.5%, E 1.5%)
Plt	215×10^9/l
Blood film	No blast cells or other abnormal blood cells
CXR	Linear atelectasis and mild hyperinflated bilateral upper zones

1. What is the most likely diagnosis?
2. How would you confirm your diagnosis?

Case 30

A 1-year-old child is hypotonic and having generalised and myoclonic seizures with comb-like rhythm activity on EEG.

Na	142 mmol/l
K	4.2 mmol/l
Bic	32 mmol/l
U	4.8 mmol/l
Cr	80 µmol/l
Ca	2.58 mmol/l
PO_4	1.47 mmol/l
Mg	0.89 mmol/l
AST	45 IU/l
ALT	40 IU/l

Leucine	925 µmol/l (65–220)
Isoleucine	198 µmol/l (26–100)
Valine	39 µmol/l (90–300)
Allo-isoleucine	190 µmol/l (1–5)
LP WCC	3
Protein	0.5 mg
Lactate	1.2 mmol/l
Alk.ph	284 IU/l
Glucose	7.1 mmol/l

1. What is the diagnosis?
2. How would you manage this child?

ANSWERS 21–30

Case 21

1. Severe aortic stenosis
2. Surgical valvotomy

Severe aortic stenosis
The child is usually extremely unwell with a low cardiac output and
congestive heart failure, cardiomegaly and pulmonary oedema.
Peripheral pulses are weak and the intensity of the murmur is low.
The pressure gradient across the stenotic valve is low because of the
low cardiac output. It is difficult to differentiate between severe aortic
stenosis and coarctation of the aorta on clinical grounds.
Echocardiography is the definitive investigation to differentiate
between these two cardiac defects.

Management
Patients with severe aortic stenosis usually present acutely at birth
with heart failure and peripheral shutdown. They can be acidotic and
severely compromised with respect to their cardio-respiratory
system. Prostaglandin infusion should be commenced to keep the
duct open. The heart failure should be treated with diuretics. Inotropic
support may be required. Digoxin is no longer used as first line
treatment for supporting the cardiovascular system. Emergency
surgical valvotomy is required for infants with critical aortic stenosis
and heart failure. Valve replacement can be done if there is a re-
stenosis, dysplastic valve or severe aortic regurgitation. Valvotomy is
indicated if patients become symptomatic with myocardial or cerebral
ischaemia, or asymptomatic with ECG changes of ST and T
abnormalities at rest or on exercise test, or if the systolic gradient on
catheterisation across the obstruction is > 50–60 mmHg. Balloon
dilatation is an alternative to surgery and the results are encouraging.

Acidosis should be corrected and fluid restricted to 40–50% of the
maintenance until the condition of the child is stable. Transfer as soon
as possible to a specialised centre is indicated for further management.

Case 22

1. Ataxia telangiectasia
2. Telangiectasia on the eyes
   Nystagmus
3. Immunoglobulins
   DNA breakage study
   Abdominal ultrasound

Ataxia telangiectasia (AT)

AT is inherited as an autosomal recessive trait and is probably due to abnormal DNA repair causing chromosomal breaks at the site of the T cell receptor gene. AT is characterised by cerebellar ataxia with progressive neurological deterioration, oculocutaneous telangiectasia, immunodeficiency with impairment of cell mediated immunity and antibody production, gonadal dysgenesis, chromosomal abnormalities, and malignant disorders. The alpha-fetoprotein and carcinoembryonic antigen are constant markers. Patients with AT are sensitive to irradiation, which causes cellular and chromosomal damage and may precipitate malignancy.

Investigations in acute cerebellar ataxia

Positive family history	Migraine, metabolic errors Dominant recurrent ataxia

↓ *negative*

Drug screen CT or MRI	Intoxication, brain tumour Haemorrhage

↓ *negative*

Lumbar puncture	Encephalitis, Miller Fisher syndrome Multiple sclerosis

↓ *negative*

HVA/VMA MRI chest and abdomen	Neuroblastoma, myoclonic encephalopathy

↓ *negative*

Glucose, lactate Amino acid analysis	Metabolic errors

↓ *negative*

Electroencephalograph	Pseudoataxia (epilepsy)

with permission from Professor Gerald M Fenichel (WB Saunders)

These are possibilities for differential diagnosis; it is not necessary for all of them to be done. A thorough history and clinical examination will be more appropriate before thinking of investigations.

Case 23

1. Haemolytic uraemic syndrome
2. Blood film
   Blood culture
   Stool culture
3. Gastroenteritis

Haemolytic uraemic syndrome (HUS)
HUS is the most common cause of acute renal failure in young children. It is characterised by the triad of micro-angiopathic anaemia, thrombocytopenia and renal failure.

Causes
The cause is not known but it can be associated with bacterial or viral infection of the gastrointestinal tract or respiratory system. HUS can be associated with SLE, malignant hypertension, and endotoxaemia.

Pathophysiology
There is endothelial injury. The micro-angiopathic anaemia results from mechanical damage to the red cells as they pass through damaged vasculature. Thrombocytopenia is due to intravascular platelet adhesion or damage.

Types of HUS
The type which is epidemic and occurs in young children following gasteroenteritis has a good prognosis. The sporadic form occurs in older children without known cause and may lead to chronic renal failure and early death.

Clinical features
HUS mostly occurs 1–2 weeks after gasteroenteritis with pallor, lethargy, dark urine, weakness and oliguria.

SLE can be associated with micro-angiopathic anaemia. Bilateral renal vein thrombosis may follow gastroenteritis. It may present with micro-angiopathic anaemia, low platelets, and acute renal failure with large kidneys—a characteristic feature of renal vein thrombosis.

Management
Renal failure can be managed conservatively, and early management with frequent peritoneal or haemodialysis will give the best chance of recovery. Plasmapheresis, anticoagulant and fresh frozen plasma are being used as part of the management; the results are not good as frequent dialysis is required.

Prognosis
The prognosis in the epidemic form is good; the sporadic form may lead to chronic renal failure. With aggressive management of acute renal failure > 90% of patients with HUS will survive the acute phase and the majority of these recover normal renal function.

Case 24

1. Check the position of the endotracheal tube (ETT)
    Chest X-ray
    Replace the nasogastric tube
2. Milk aspiration

Milk aspiration is usually due to an absent gag reflex or swallowing incoordination. It may also follow GOR or injury to lower cranial nerves (brainstem lesions).

Neonatal hypotonia can present as:

↓	↓
Reflexes absent	*Reflexes present*
↓	↓
Anterior horn cell defect	Neuromuscular junction defect
Peripheral nerve neuropathy	(myasthenia gravis)
Myopathies	Central nervous system
	malformation, haemorrhage
	Hypoxic ischaemic encephalopathy,
	drug intoxications
	Mixed origin (hypothyroidism,
	Prader–Willi syndrome,
	Zellweger syndrome)
	Trisomy 21
	Connective tissue abnormality,
	(Marfan, Ehlers–Danlos syndrome)
	Benign congenital hypotonia

The gene defect of myotonic dystrophy is located by an unstable fragment of deoxyribonucleic acid detected on chromosome 19 in all patients, and the size of the fragment correlates with the disease severity. Prenatal diagnosis can be informative in more than 90% of affected cases. Genetic counselling is required.

Case 25

1. Precocious puberty
2. Congenital adrenal hyperplasia (CAH)
3. Serum electrolytes
17-hydroxyprogesterone
Karyotyping
Abdominal ultrasound

Precocious puberty
Precocious puberty can be gonadotropin dependent or independent.

	Gonadotropin dependent	Gonadotropin independent
Sex	More common in females	M:F 1:1
Bone age	Advanced	Advanced
Stature	Short	Short
LH	Detected in 50–70% of cases	Low
GnRH stimulation test	Response LH > FSH	No response
Estradiol	Low in early stages Boys > girls	High in girls—not always if cause is adrenal
Pituitary	Normal on imaging	May be abnormal on imaging
Ovaries	Large on US	Large
Uterus	Large	Large
Treatment	IM long-acting GnRH	

Treatment in gonadotropin dependent cases will decrease the rate of growth and osseous maturation. The height can be predicted easily and will be approximately 1 SD below the midparental height. In girls breast development may regress in Tanner stage II–III and may show no changes or may increase in Tanner III–IV. Pubic hair growth will not progress and the size of the ovaries and uterus is reduced. The sum of sex hormone concentration, including LH and FSH, decreases to prepubertal levels if treatment is effective.

Case 26

1. Muscle pain
2. Urine for myoglobulinuria
   Electromyography (EMG)
   Serum lactate and serum ammonia
3. Myopathies
   Glycogen storage disease
   Fatty acid oxidation defect

Muscle pain and cramps
Strenuous exercise and excessive loss of electrolytes and fluids may cause muscle pain and cramps. It is characterised on EMG by the repetitive firing of normal motor unit potentials. The cramps will often resolve by stretching the muscle. Partially denervated muscle is more susceptible to cramps during exercise and sleep. Cramps during exercise can occur in patients with disorders of muscle energy metabolism which are difficult to detect on EMG.

Children can present with muscle pain which is not resolved by stretching, and the muscles are not in a spasmodic state. These are not symptoms of neuromuscular disease; the symptoms can be relieved by mild analgesia.

An approach to diagnosis in a child with muscle cramps or pain
Forearm ischaemic exercise test.

Place the blood pressure cuff around the arm. Insert an indwelling catheter in the antecubital vein and obtain a sample for lactate, ammonia and CK 10 minutes before exercise. Inflate the cuff 20 mmHg above systolic pressure and ask the patient to squeeze a hand dynamometer 40 times in 1 minute and then 2 times per second for 1 minute. Release the cuff pressure and collect blood for lactate, ammonia and CK. Repeat this test at 3, 5, 10 and 20 minutes.

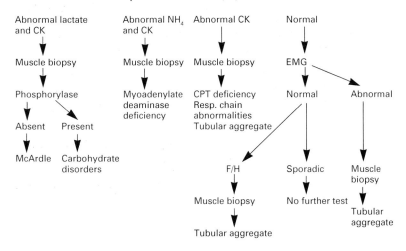

With kind permission from Gerald M Fenichel (Clinical Paediatric Neurology)

Case 27

1. Large amplitude slow periodic complexes occurring every 3–4 seconds
2. Sub-acute sclerosing panencephalitis (SSPE)
3. Poor. Measles vaccine at 13–15 months of age (MMR)

Sub-acute sclerosing panencephalitis (SSPE)
This is the most common chronic encephalitis in children. It is caused by the measles virus following infection in the first two years of life.

Pathogenesis
The pathogenesis is unclear; there is no immunodeficiency. Recent work suggests that there is a mutation in the genes coding for M and F viral proteins.

On microscopic examination there is vascular cuffing by mononuclear cells, neuronal loss and marked fibrillary glial proliferation. The incidence of the disease is 1 per 1 000 000 cases of measles.

EEG
The characteristic EEG abnormality may be observed before the clinical features. EEG shows large amplitude slow periodic complexes occurring every 3–4 seconds.

Clinical features
Children usually present with a history of loss of skills, clumsiness and drop attacks. Seizures occur in 30% of cases. The disease progress is slow in typical cases with marked changes in personality and intellectual deterioration. Involuntary movement appears within 2–4 months in the form of bilateral myoclonic jerks. Extrapyramidal or pyramidal dysfunction or both appear before the terminal stage which is characterised by a progressive unresponsiveness, increasing tone, dementia, and decerebrate rigidity. This is also associated with respiratory difficulties and autonomic impairment, and patients die within 1–3 years after the start of the clinical manifestation.

Diagnosis
The CSF contains no cells and has a normal protein level with slightly elevated gammaglobulins, mainly IgG with oligoclonal bands. Specific antibodies against measles are high in both CSF and serum. CT and MRI scans are normal. Steroids, interferon and antiviral drugs have been used as a therapeutic trial without benefit.

Case 28

1. Chronic liver disease with portal hypertension
2. Liver biopsy
   Portal vein Doppler ultrasound

Auto-immune liver disease (chronic active hepatitis—CAH)
Liver function is abnormal with raised AST, ALT, and gammaglobulin. The PT and PTT are prolonged. The IgG is raised and the ESR high.

Auto-immune hepatitis is a non-infectious chronic active hepatitis. The non-organic specific antibody, e.g. antinuclear antibody, antimitochondrial antibody, smooth muscle antibody, liver and kidney microsomal antibody, will be high. CAH occurs in children between 2 and 14 years of age. The symptoms are usually vague and the child may present with hepatomegaly or abnormal liver enzyme tests. Sometimes the presentation is with arthralgia, bleeding problems, acne, cushingoid features and fever. Abrupt onset with jaundice, abdominal pain and ascites can occur. Liver cirrhosis with varicose veins and encephalopathy is a late feature which indicates a poor prognosis.

Investigations
Needle liver biopsy is the confirmatory test after correction of coagulopathy. The histology is piecemeal necrosis, and plasma cell infiltration is the cardinal feature. Another investigation which may be helpful is the phenomenon of auto-antibodies. Lupus erythematosus cells occur in some 15% of cases.

Treatment
Corticosteroid therapy with or without low doses of azathioprine improves the clinical, biochemical and histological features in most patients with auto-immune chronic active hepatitis. More than 75% will respond to corticosteroid therapy. Progress to cirrhosis may occur despite a good response to therapy. Corticosteroids are not effective in HBsAg positive cases.

Case 29

1. Whooping cough
2. Serology and pernasal swab for *Bordetella pertussis*

Whooping cough
The persistence of cough with CXR changes and lymphocytosis on differential blood count should alert the clinician to look for *Bordetella pertussis* as a cause.

Humans are the only known host to *Bordetella pertussis*, which multiplies only on ciliated epithelium. The incubation period is 6–20 days. Transplacental maternal antibody does not protect newborn babies for a longer period.

Clinical features
There are different stages of the disease:

- The catarrhal stage lasts 1–2 weeks and presents like an upper respiratory tract infection.
- The paroxysmal stage lasts 2–4 weeks and is characterised by episodes of spasmodic coughing followed by a sudden whoop as air is drawn into the lungs. Vomiting, cyanosis, epistaxis and seizures may occur. The coughing episodes increase in severity and number.
- The convalescent stage lasts 1–2 weeks with paroxysmal episodes of coughing which decrease in intensity and frequency.

Investigations
There is an absolute lymphocytosis > 20 000. The chest X-ray will show air trapping, bronchial wall thickening and hyperinflation of the lungs. Measurement of a rise in antibody titres and culture of

Bordetella pertussis can be done but it takes a long time to get a positive result. Pernasal swabs for culture and direct fluorescent antibody can be done later to confirm the presence of infection.

Management
Expert nursing with fluids and nutritional support is essential during the paroxysmal phase. Erythromycin given for 2 weeks reduces the period of infectivity. Inhaled steroids are being used by some paediatricians. Vaccination should be given; it is contraindicated if there is a bad reaction to the first dose, intractable epilepsy or progressive encephalopathy. In cases of febrile convulsion, neurological disorders and progressive neurological disorders, vaccination can be given after consultation with the paediatric neurologist.

Case 30

1. Maple syrup urine disease
2. Low protein diet
    Anticonvulsant
    Genetic counselling

Maple syrup urine disease (MSUD)
MSUD can be suspected if a neonate or infant presents with metabolic acidosis, generalised clonic seizures, vomiting and muscle rigidity.

There is an increase in plasma leucine, isoleucine and valine amino acid levels. This is due to reduced activity of branched-chain keto-acid decarboxylase. The inheritance is autosomal recessive. The severe form manifests in the early days of life with severe neurological symptoms, acidosis and hyperammonaemia; death occurs early in life. Clearance of accumulated toxic amino acids by peritoneal dialysis and halting the catabolic state by providing enough calories via total parenteral nutrition is vital for children who present with acute symptoms.

The mild form is difficult to recognise and may present during infection or any other illness with acidosis and lethargy. Restricted diet control in the form of a low protein intake is necessary. Synthetic branched amino acids (leucine, isoleucine and valine) are indicated in moderate and mild forms which are not responding to thiamine therapy. Mental and neurological problems are a common sequel.

Prenatal diagnosis is available and genetic counselling is recommended in all cases.

Infants or children with organic acidaemia may present with lack of feeding, vomiting, acidosis, dehydration and neutropenia. They may be ketotic and have skin manifestations. This is a common feature of multiple carboxylase deficiency. If there is no skin manifestation but a characteristic odour, it could be either MSUD or isovaleric acidaemia (sweaty feet). If there is no odour there may be other causes such as methylmalonic acidaemia and propionic acidaemia.

Case 31

A 2-month-old infant presented with central cyanosis which was not persistent. Cardiac catheterisation was performed.

	O_2 saturation	Mean pressure (mmHg)
SVC	44%	
IVC	56%	
RA	85%	
RV	84%	79
PA	84%	50
PV	93%	10
LA	73%	
LV	84%	12

1. What is the most likely diagnosis?

Case 32

A 2-year-old boy presented with a 7-day history of ulcerated skin lesions. No lymphadenopathy was noted. He had a history of frequent otitis media. His weight was below the 3rd centile. There were no tonsils on examination.

Hb	11 g/dl
WCC	$5 \times 10^9/l$ (N 1.0)
Plt	$332 \times 10^9/l$

Blood culture revealed pseudomonas.

1. What are the most likely diagnoses?
2. Give one alternative diagnosis.

He was treated with antibiotics. His white cell count rose to $19 \times 10^9/l$ with a neutrophilia. Unfortunately he was admitted two weeks later with pseudomonas osteomyelitis.

IgG	< 1 g/l (6–15)
IgA	0.5 g/l (0.5–4)
IgM	0.2 g/l (0.2–4)

3. What is the diagnosis?

Case 33

A 10-month-old infant presented with puffiness of his face. He was treated with antibiotics for URTI. Two days before presentation, a macular rash appeared on his thigh and trunk.

Na	138 mmol/l
K	4.5 mmol/l
U	9.2 mmol/l
Cr	47 µmol/l
Alb	19 g/l
Hb	12.7 g/dl
WCC	13.8×10^9/l
Plt	450×10^9/l
ESR	95 mm/h
ASOT	Normal
Urine	
Na	21 mmol/l
K	85 mmol/l
Ur	330 mmol/l
Urine output	3 ml/kg/h
Protein	++++
Blood	+

Renal biopsy showed a diffuse increase in mesangial cells and matrix with IgM and C3 deposit.

1.   What is the diagnosis?
2.   What are the three most common histopathological changes causing this illness?
3.   What is the prognosis?

Case 34

A 21-month-old infant presented with a history of vomiting. She had been diagnosed as having tonsillitis and had been treated with erythromycin for 5 days. Her vomiting increased progressively and her mother took her to hospital. All of her mother's brothers had died soon after birth.

She was irritable and banging her head on the bed. She showed abnormal posturing, and brisk reflexes with extensor plantars.

Na	138 mmol/l
K	3.8 mmol/l
U	2.7 mmol/l
Cr	52 µmol/l
Glucose	5 mmol/l
Arterial blood gas	
pH	7.42
PCO_2	3.7 kPa
PO_2	60 kPa
Be	1.2

LP normal; pyruvate and lactate normal.

1.   What is the next blood test you would do?
2.   What are the underlying causes?

Case 35

This 4 year old failed his hearing test at school.

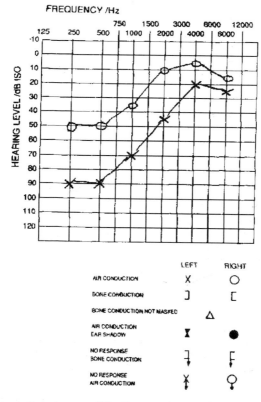

1. What are the abnormalities?
2. What is the underlying cause?

Case 36

A 2-week-old boy presented with a history of lethargy, sweating and breathlessness. He had been vomiting for the last 6 hours at a rate of 6 vomits/h.

Na	117 mmol/l
K	7.5 mmol/l
U	16.1 mmol/l
Cr	70 µmol/l
Ammonia	10 mmol/l
Glucose	3.4 mmol/l

LFT and FBC are normal. Urine culture is sterile.

1. What is the diagnosis?
2. What other physical sign will you look for?
3. What is the immediate management?

Case 37

A 2-day-old infant had apnoea attacks and floppiness, and needed ventilation for 17 days. Since he has been off the ventilator he has frequently had the hiccups.

Plasma AA	Normal, apart from elevated glycerine at 597 (100–330 μmol/l)
Plasma NH_4	80 μmol/l (< 200)
Plasma lactate	2.1 mmol/l (2–4)
Plasma electrolytes and urea	Normal, no ketonuria
CSF lactate	2.1 mmol/l
CSF/plasma ratio for glycerine	0.35

1. What is the diagnosis?
2. What other investigation will you ask for?

Case 38

A child can draw a circle, cross, square and triangle. This is what she draws at school.

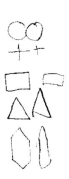 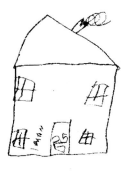

1. What is the nearest age you can suggest?
2. Will she be able to know her name, surname, address and home telephone number?
3. How would you test her vision?

Case 39

These are the results of CSF analysis from a 3-year-old child who was referred to Casualty by his desperate GP. He has been treated for tonsillitis with erythromycin for 7 days without improvement.

Lumbar puncture revealed:

Pressure	18 mmHg (8–10)
WC	800 polymorphs
Protein	6.5 g
Glucose	1.6 mmol/l
Gram stain	Negative

1. What is the most likely diagnosis?
2. What further investigations are required?

Case 40

A 12-year-old girl has a history of headache and limb pain. Two weeks ago she had chicken pox. There is evidence of healing chicken pox lesions. Reflexes from the lower limbs are absent. There is neck pain with normal muscle power.

Hb	13.3 g/dl
WCC	8×10^9/l (N 48%, L 44%, M 3.55%, E 2.3%, B 2.2%)
Plt	425×10^9/l
ESR	15 mm/h
CSF	
Protein	3 g
WCC	7 (100% lymphocytes)
Sugar	2.8 mmol

- Nerve conduction study: there is latency for motor part
- MRI head and spine normal.

1. What is the most likely diagnosis?
2. Name three procedures which you would perform as a part of the management?

ANSWERS 31–40

Case 31

1. Total anomalous pulmonary venous drainage with ASD (TAPVD + ASD)

Total anomalous pulmonary venous drainage
The saturation in the RA and RV is higher than that on the left side of the heart, which suggests that the pulmonary veins join the systemic venous system before entering the right atrium. The pulmonary

artery pressure is high as pulmonary hypertension is commonly associated with TAPVD. The prognosis is poor unless surgery is performed early.

The pulmonary veins may enter the RA, superior or inferior vena cava, ductus venosum or hepatic veins. The condition is usually associated with an ASD and can be divided into supra- or infra-diaphragmatic according to the entry of the pulmonary veins into the venous system. In the newborn, it usually presents with intermittent cyanosis, tachypnoea and a systolic murmur. In cases where there is severe obstruction of the pulmonary venous return, the baby will present with cyanosis and no murmurs. If there is a left to right shunt at the arterial or ventricular level, patients usually present with congestive cardiac failure in early life and pulmonary hypertension. ECG will show right ventricular hypertrophy (V4R,V1) and a tall spiked P wave. CXR will show the characteristic 'snow man' or 'figure of eight' shape.

Case 32

1. X-linked hypogammaglobulinaemia
   Leukocyte adhesion deficiency (LAD)
   Chronic granulomatous disease (CGD)
2. Severe combined immune deficiency syndrome (SCID)
3. X-linked hypogammaglobulinaemia

X-linked hypogammaglobulinaemia

Disease	Clinical criteria	Functional defect	Pathogenesis	Inheritance
Leukocyte adhesion deficiency (LAD)	Delayed separation of umbilical cord Skin infection and gingivitis Deep abscess and osteomyelitis	Decrease in phagocytosis and adherence	Absence of adhesion CD11a,b,c due to defect in CD18 on neutrophils, lymphocytes	Autosomal recessive
Chronic granulomatous disease (CGD)	Repeated infection with catalase-negative bacteria Granuloma formation	Decreased oxidative metabolism, decreased microbiocidal activity	Lack of cytochromes	X-linked recessive AR
X-linked hypogamma-globulinaemia	Repeated bacterial infection	Panhypogamma-globulinaemia Reduced antibody activity Isohaemagglutinin not detected Lymphocyte function normal	B cell absent T cell normal	X-linked recessive

Case 33

1. Nephrotic syndrome
2. Minimal change glomerulonephritis (MCGN)
   Focal segmental glomerulosclerosis (FSGN)
   Mesangial proliferative glomerulonephritis (MPGN)
3. Very good

Nephrotic syndrome (NS)

The proteinuria and oedema are characteristic features of NS. NS, in 90% of all cases, is idiopathic. On renal biopsy, 85% of these show minimal changes, 10% focal sclerosis and 5% mesangial proliferative glomerulonephritis. Other causes include SLE, bronchiectasis, etc. NS is characterised by increased glomerular capillary wall permeability to protein of more than 2 g/day. Oedema appears when the serum albumin level is <25 g/l. There is also an increase in serum lipids (triglycerides and cholesterol) and lipoproteins. The syndrome suggests several diseases having similar clinical manifestations.

Histopathology

	Biopsy	Immunofluorescence	Response to steroids
MCGN	Minimal increase in mesangial cells and matrix	Negative	95%
FSGN	Majority of glomeruli are normal. Focal mesangial proliferation and scarring	Negative	20%
MPGN	Diffuse increase in mesangial cells and matrix	IgM and C3	50–60%

Complications

The incidence of infection increases because the immunoglobulin level is reduced, oedema is a rich medium, there is protein deficiency, bactericidal activity of the leukocytes is decreased, and there is hypovolaemia and loss of complement in urine which reduces the opsonisation of certain bacteria (e.g. pneumococci).

Another complication is the increased incidence of arterial and venous thrombosis which may be due to decreased levels of antithrombin III and an increase in platelet aggregation.

Management

Remission can be achieved by prednisolone 60 mg/m²/day until the urine becomes free, trace or 1+ on dipstick of protein. Daily prednisolone is maintained until the urine is protein free or negative for 3 days, then the dose is changed to 40 mg/m²/24 h on alternate days for 28 days. It is then stopped gradually over the next 3–4 weeks. Every relapse is treated with the same regimen. Cyclophosphamide and cyclosporine can be used where there is resistance to steroid. Very rarely NS can be carried into adult life.

Case 34

1. Ammonia level
2. Urea cycle defect

Hyperammonaemia
The most likely diagnosis in this case is a *urea cycle defect* due to ornithine transcarbamylase deficiency. Male patients usually present in the first few days of life with an encephalopathy-like illness and die after a few days if appropriate treatment is not given. It is an X-linked dominant disorder.

Female carriers may have a mild form of the disease. The onset occurs during high protein intake, infection or starvation. Death may occur following a coma with hyperammonaemia. Mental development is usually normal. There is a marked increase of urine orotic acid which differentiates OTC from other forms of urea cycle defect.

Reye's syndrome
Transient neonatal hyperammonaemia
Hyperornithinaemia, hyperammonaemia.

Homocitrullinuria (*HHH syndrome*). There is developmental delay with spastic quadriplegia as the child grows older.

Secondary hyperammonaemia:

- Liver disease—acute liver failure
- Lactic acidaemia
- Ketotic hyperglycinaemia
- Neonatal glutaric aciduria type II
- Fatty oxidation defect
- Valproic acid toxicity

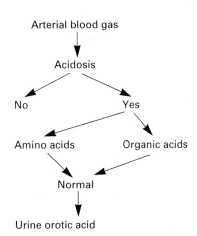

Management of acute hyperammonemia is with low protein (0.25 g/kg/day); phenylacetate, sodium benzoate and arginine should be given as soon as possible, and if there is no improvement dialysis should be considered. If there is a good result, then maintain the above regimen. All patients should be supplied with an emergency kit for acute hyperammonaemia treatment.

Case 35

1. Bilateral conductive hearing loss
2. Otitis media

Methods of checking hearing by patient age group

- Neonates can be tested using the acoustic response cradle. This is an automatic microprocessor controlled device used to detect hearing response against a background of spontaneous activity. In high risk groups brainstem auditory evoked response (BSAER) is the method of choice for testing hearing in neonates.
- Distraction audiometry is used as a screening test at 7–8 months of age.
- Toy discrimination test. A normal child can discriminate the verbal toy stimuli at 40 dB at 3 feet. This can be applied to age 2–5 years.
- Audiometry can be applied to any child over the age of 5 years.
- Tympanometry can be applied at any age.
- Brainstem auditory evoked response (BSAER) can be used from an early age, as a response first appears at a conceptional age of 26–27 weeks.

Methods adapted for screening hearing in babies include respiratory audiometry, observation audiometry, visual reinforcement audiometry, and play audiometry. None of these is entirely reliable and examination should be repeated, especially if no response to the sound is obtained. BSAER is again preferred if it is available.

Case 36

1. Congenital adrenal hyperplasia (CAH)
2. Skin pigmentation
3. Intravenous dextrose saline fluid, hydrocortisone and intensive support care

Congenital adrenal hyperplasia (CAH)
The commonest enzyme deficiency associated with CAH is 21-hydroxylase deficiency.

Clinical features
Newborn male infants commonly do not show any abnormality (occasionally a Caucasian newborn will have a dark scrotum). Newborn female infants show virilisation as a result of exposure to DHA, testosterone and androsterone. Female infants are usually born

with ambiguous genitalia. They may present with salt loss crisis by the age of 3–4 weeks. Salt loss crises can occur in both male and female infants.

Investigation of ambiguous genitalia

Test	Comment
1. Karyotype	1. Preliminary results available within 48 hours
2. 17-OHP in plasma or blood spot	2. Placental 17-OHP may interfere in first 24 hours Overlap with the raised levels in sick or preterm infants is rare
3. Electrolytes: a. Plasma K$^+$ b. Plasma Na$^+$ c. Urinary Na$^+$	3. a. Increased. Often precedes fall in Na$^+$ b. Decreased c. Increased
4. Plasma testosterone	4. Frequently within adult male range
5. Plasma renin activity (PRA)	5. Increased. Sensitive index of salt depletion but result seldom available immediately
6. Urinary steroid metabolites	6. Confirms site of block, especially in the rare enzyme defects
7. Pelvic ultrasound	7. Reassures parents about normal female internal genitalia
8. Sinogram	8. Occasionally required to show internal genital anatomy

Permission has been granted by Professor Ieuan A Hughes to use this material

Cloning of the gene by DNA analysis can be done to determine carrier status as well as enabling prenatal diagnosis to be carried out.

Surgical correction can be done at the age of puberty in girls.

About 5% of CAH is due to 11 β-hydroxylase deficiency. These cases can present like 21OH deficiency but with high blood pressure.

Treatment
Cortisol replacement (hydrocortisone 12–25 mg/m^2/day in two doses). It is necessary to monitor growth and virilisation as well as 17-OHP and testosterone levels. Patients also require salt and aldosterone replacement (salt—up to 5 mmol/kg/day; fludrocortisone— 100–200 µg/day in divided doses) and their blood pressure should be monitored as well as plasma renin activity and electrolytes.

Case 37

1.   Non-ketotic hyperglycinaemia
2.   Brain MRI and EEG

	Ketotic hyperglycinaemia (organic acidaemias)	Non-ketotic hyperglycinaemia
Inheritance	AR	AR
Ammonia	High	Normal
Ketoacidosis	Abnormal	Normal
Glucose	Low	Normal
Lactate	High	Normal
Glycine	High	Normal
Neutrophils	Low	Normal
Thrombocytes	Low	Normal
CSF/plasma glycine ratio	Normal	Increased
Seizures	Multiple seizures type	Myoclonic
EEG	Generalised activity	Suppression-burst, hypsarrhythmia
MRI	Non-specific changes	Progressive cerebral atrophy and demyelination of supratentorial white matter

Case 38

1. 4½ years
2. Yes
3. STYCAR letter test

By 4 years of age, a child can draw a man with a head, trunk, two extremities and clothing. He or she starts to have a language at the social function level and to choose sentences and engage in conversations. There is more involvement with other children for various activities.

Visual assessment in different age groups
- Ask parents about any problems with vision in the child.
- Eye examination with examination of the fundi in all age groups.
- In neonates and younger infants, observe the child to see if he/she can fix on and follow an object or human face at a distance of 3 metres.
- Below 2½ years by using 10 white balls of varying sizes (from one-eighth to 2½ inches in diameter) which are rolled on a dark strip horizontally to the line of the infant's gaze, some 3 metres from the child. It is important to note that visualization of even the smallest ball does not mean the vision is perfect.
- The STYCAR (by Sheridan) letter test can be started from 2½ years of age by matching the letters as follows. Present a single letter of decreasing size at 3 metres. The child has a key card which has either five (2½–3½ years), seven (3½–4½ years) or nine (5–7 years) capital letters on it.
- The Key Picture Test is similar to the STYCAR letter test but it uses pictures and can be used by some children as young as 18 months.

- Snellen charts can be used from the age of 7 years.
- Visual evoked response (VER) to flashes is an excellent technique to demonstrate the integrity of the visual pathways without patient cooperation (Baker 1995). By the age of 3 months the morphology and latency of the visual evoked responses are relatively mature, but interpretation may still be difficult.

Case 39

1. Tuberculous meningitis
2. Ziehl–Neelsen stain for CSF
   Chest X-ray

TB meningitis
The high CSF presssure, protein and low sugar will be in favour of TB meningitis. Partially treated meningitis can present like this but the CSF protein will not be high, nor will CSF glucose be very low. The other condition which may present with high CSF protein is spinal abscess but CSF pressure is high and CSF sugar normal.

Diagnosis
Tuberculous meningitis is the most likely diagnosis and will be the first on the list. The tests which should be done on CSF are a Ziehl–Neelsen stain and CSF culture for mycobacterium using Löwenstein–Jensen medium, the results of which will be available in 6 weeks. A Mantoux test using 0.1 ml of tuberculin purified protein (PPD) of 1–1000 intradermally on the upper third of the flexor aspect of the forearm can be read after 72 hours. A positive result consists of transverse induration of at least 5 mm diameter; 0-4 mm induration is negative, 4–15 mm is equivalent to Heaf grade 2, and 15 mm or more is strongly positive and equivalent to Heaf grade 3–4. The latter is indicative of TB infection, even if the clinical signs are not convincing, and treatment should be started. 1–10 000 concentration can be used in patients strongly suspected of having TB or tuberculin sensitive patients. ELISA is used but its use is not widespread. Polymerase chain reaction (PCR) is more reliable but not available in many countries where tuberculous meningitis is common. Chest X-ray should be done as well as CT brain scan to exclude tuberculoma.

In patients with immunosuppressive disease or on immunosuppressive therapy, tuberculosis should be excluded as early as possible as the incidence of tuberculosis has been increasing in the last few years.

Complications of TB meningitis include cranial nerve palsy, hydrocephalus, seizures, tuberculoma and SIADH.

Case 40

1. Guillain–Barré syndrome
2. Lung function
   Peak expiratory flow rate
   Blood pressure

Guillain–Barré syndrome

The history of headache and muscle pain following a viral infection will be difficult to diagnose unless you have done another investigation. The investigation at this stage will be lumbar puncture.

- Blood for virology titres (polio, adenovirus, enterovirus), mycoplasma IgM, and *Borrelia burgdorferi* IgM
- Nerve conduction study
- Urine for myoglobinuria
- CT or MRI of brain and spine.

In this case the CSF shows high protein and normal sugar with low WCC. All of these make Guillain–Barré syndrome the most likely diagnosis.

Myeloencephalitis can present like this at the beginning but focal neurological signs with upper and lower motor tract signs will appear later.

Guillain–Barré syndrome is a post-infectious polyneuropathy that causes demyelination in the anterior horn cells. This causes rapidly evolving flaccid paralysis starting at the lower extremities and progressively involving the upper limbs. The respiratory muscles and face may be involved. The autonomic nerve system may also be involved and present with labile blood pressure, bradycardia and urinary retention.

Muscle pain and tenderness is common in children. The child may refuse to walk due to pain and may complain of paraesthesia. Bulbar involvement occurs in half of the patients, and some may require respiratory support by ventilator. In patients with bulbar involvement, lung function assessment is indicated with frequent measurement of vital capacity. The nerve conduction study will show marked reduction in motor velocity and sensory velocity may be low. The EMG will show acute denervation of the muscle.

Management

The current treatment is by using intravenous immunoglobulin of 2 g/kg infused over 18 hours; this is more effective than a 5-day course of IVIG. Most of the patients recover; a few are left with chronic problems, in particular those patients with extensive autonomic system involvement. The course of the disease varies from a few weeks to over 6 months.

Case 41

A newborn baby started to fit at the age of 3 hours. The mother required IV fluids of 5% dextrose for 12 hours up to 150 ml/kg.

Glucose	3.4 mmol/l
Blood, urine, and CSF cultures after 48 hours with no growth	
Ca	2.21 mmol/l
Mg	0.90 mmol/l
PO_4	1.21 mmol/l
Hb	17.3 g/dl
WCC	6.7×10^9/l
Plt	195×10^9/l
Urine	
WCC	1
RBCs	0 epithelial cast + Gram stain
CSF	
WCC	7
RBCs	10
Protein	0.34 g
Glucose	2.1 mmol/l
No organism	

1. What is the most likely cause of the fits?
2. How can they be prevented?

Case 42

These are the results of cardiac catheterisation performed on a 7-month-old boy with a history of cyanosis.

Saturation	89–94% on oxymeter
Pressure	
AO (D)	122/54 (85) D/S (M)
AO (A)	118/54 (81)
LV	121/9
LA	14/4 (9)
RA	5
RVO	97/2
RV body	112/9
Left-sided aortic arch on echocardiography	

1. What is the diagnosis?
2. What are the risk factors at this stage?

Case 43

A 1-year-old child had a history of failure to thrive. Birth weight was 4 kg, and he had been breastfed for 6 months. At the age of one year his weight was only 8 kg.

Hb	11.2 g/dl
WCC	6.2 × 10⁹/l
Plt	180 × 10⁹/l

Hb   11.2 g/dl
WCC   6.2 × 10^9/l
Plt   180 × 10^9/l
Blood film   Hypochromia, anisocytosis and acanthocytosis
X-ray of wrist shows evidence of rickets
Serum cholesterol   0.7 mmol/l
Stool shows fat globules

1.   What is the diagnosis and what is the mode of inheritance?
2.   How would the diagnosis be confirmed?
3.   What other clinical signs may be present?

Case 44

This is the result of a procedure carried out on an 18-month-old girl with prenatal diagnosis of right renal dilatation (12 mm) and abnormal left kidney.

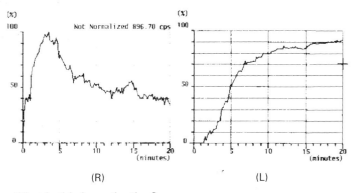

(R)   (L)

1.   What is this investigation?
2.   Is it abnormal?

Case 45

A 7-year-old child presented with status epilepticus. The seizures terminated with emergency treatment. These are the investigation results. Of note in the past is a history of pica.

Hb   7.1 g/dl
WCC   8.3 × 10^9/l
Plt   175 × 10^9/l

Ca	2.23 mmol/l
Glucose	5.2 mmol/l
Na	121 mmol/l
K	4.9 mmol/l
U	3.4 µmol/l
CSF	
WCC	4
RBCs	40
No organism seen	
Protein	0.23 mg/l
Glucose	3.1 mmol/l
Urine	
Protein	+++
Amino acid	+++

1. What is the most likely diagnosis?
2. What is the cause of the low sodium level and how would you manage this problem ?
3. List further appropriate investigations to aid diagnosis.

Case 46

A 10-year-old boy presented with a history of generalised pain, high fever and aches for the last 2 days. Both liver and spleen are palpable measuring 3 cm.

He lives near a lake and has been swimming in this lake from time to time during the summer holiday. He is from the Middle East. The following results were obtained:

Hb	11.5 g/dl
WCC	3.2×10^9/l (N 40%, polys 70%)
Plt	200×10^9/l
Na	133 mmol/l
K	3.5 mmol/l
U	7.5 mmol/l
Cr	80 µmol/l
CSF	
Glucose	4.1 mmol/l
No organisms	
Protein	30 mg/l

1. What is the most likely diagnosis?
2. Give one test to confirm your diagnosis.

Case 47

A 6-month-old infant was referred with failure to thrive. He has been constipated since birth. His milk intake is 120 ml every 2 hours. He wakes during the night crying but he will go back to sleep after a feed of 120 ml of milk.

Na	131 mmol/l
Hb	12 g/dl
K	2.7 mmol/l
WCC	7.5×10^9/l
Cl-	85 mmol/l
Plt	190×10^9/l
Cr	45 μmol/l
Protein	30 g/l
U	3.9 mmol/l
Urine	
Na	10 mmol/l
K	60 mmol/l
pH	7.50
U	200 mmol/l
HCO_3^-	30 kPa
pH	6.2

1.   What is the differential diagnosis?
2.   Which investigation will aid diagnosis?
3.   What is the most likely diagnosis and what is your treatment?

Case 48

A 5-month-old boy was found by his mother suffering a generalised fit which lasted 20 minutes. This persisted on arrival at the Emergency Department. His bedside blood glucose level was unrecordable. 10% dextrose was administered intravenously at a rate of 8 mg/kg/min. 30 minutes later his blood glucose level was 2 mmol/l. Hypoglycaemia persisted despite an infusion of 12 mg/kg/min of 10% glucose. A laboratory glucose analysis revealed hypoglycaemia.

1.   What three further investigations are indicated?
2.   List three differential diagnoses.

Case 49

A 10-year-old girl was brought to the Accident & Emergency Department by her mother as she had developed worsening swelling around her eyes and ankles during the afternoon. Her father had died suddenly from upper respiratory obstruction of uncertain aetiology ten years previously.

Urine	No protein or blood
Hb	13 g/dl
WCC	8.3×10^9/
Plt	265×10^9/l
Na	139 mmol/l
K	4.2 mmol/l
U	3.1 mmol/l

Cr	35 µmol/l
ALT	9 IU/l
Alk.ph	12 IU/l
Bili	6 µmol/l
Alb	35 g/l
T protein	70 g/l
IgE	210 g/l
C3, C4	normal

1. What is the diagnosis?
2. What is the underlying problem?
3. Outline your management of this girl.

Case 50

A 6-year-old girl presents with purpura. She has shotty palpable occipital and left cervical lymph nodes. Examination of her limbs reveals an absent right thumb. She suffers with mild mental retardation.

1. What is the diagnosis?
2. What other physical signs would you look for?
3. What investigations are indicated?

ANSWERS 41–50

Case 41

1. Hyponatraemia secondary to hypervolaemia and oxytocin
2. Maintenance fluid to mother
   Oxytocin only during second stage

Hyponatraemia (Na < 130 mmol/l)

Aetiology

Loss of sodium in excess of water	Gain of water in excess of sodium
External loss	SIADH
Gastro-intestinal—diarrhoea	Renal failure
Skin—excessive sweating	Excessive water intake
Third space losses—burns	Oedematous states
Renal salt loss	
Renal—RTA, diuretic therapy	
Non-renal CAH/Addison's	

Investigation of hyponatraemia

Aetiology	Loss of water in excess of Na		Gain of water in excess of sodium	
Investigation	External loss	Renal salt loss	Oedematous states	SIADH
Volume	Reduced	Increased	Reduced	Reduced
Urine Na	< 20 mmol/l	> 20 mmol/l	< 20 mmol/l	> 20 mmol/l
Urine osmo.	> 500 mosmol/l	Isotonic	> 500 mosmol/l	Hyperosmolar
Plasma urea	Increased	Increased	Normal or increased	Normal or reduced
Plasma osmo.	Reduced	Reduced	Reduced	Reduced

Case 42

1. Fallot's tetralogy
2. Cyanotic spells
   Embolism
   Infection

Fallot's tetralogy (FT)

Cardiac catheterisation and angiography are still performed before or during surgery to provide more information. The ECG in tetralogy of Fallot will show right ventricular hypertrophy and right axis deviation. Echocardiography is the diagnostic procedure with evaluation of pulmonary artery pressure. About 20–30% of patients with FT will show a right aortic arch. Chest X-ray will show oligaemic lung.

Treatment is divided into palliative surgery and total correction. Palliative surgery can be done after birth if the infant presents with severe FT. The procedure is the Blalock–Taussig operation. Total correction is usually done after the first year of life, depending on the size of the child and the symptoms.

Treatment of cyanotic spells:
- 100% oxygen via facial mask
- IV propranolol and then maintenance
- Watch for side effects in asthmatic and low blood sugar
- Correct metabolic acidosis with colloids or bicarbonate
- Check haematocrit, haemoglobin, and clotting

Case 43

1. Abetalipoprotinaemia
2. Blood protein lipase enzyme
3. Ataxia and retinitis pigmentosa

Abetalipoproteinaemia

Clinical features
Abetalipoproteinaemia is an autosomal recessive disorder resulting from lack of synthesis of apoprotein B which is essential for the

formation of low density lipoprotein (LDL), very low density lipoprotein (VLDL) and chylomicrons. The homozygous will have no chylomicrons, LDL and VLDL. The cholesterol level is < 1.3 mmol/l and triglycerides < 0.2 mmol/l. The heterozygous have no clinical or biochemical abnormality.

The patient presents with features of fat malabsorption and diarrhoea. Bleeding may occur due to vitamin K malabsorption and there may be signs and symptoms of malabsorption of other fat soluble vitamins. Acanthocytosis (spiky red cells) is always present from birth but is not pathognomonic.

Diagnosis
The diagnosis can be confirmed by lipid electrophoresis which will show absence of LDL.
Evoked retinography (ERG) is extinguished, the serum cholesterol level is low, EMG shows denervation and conduction velocities are diminished.

Management and prognosis
Retinitis pigmentosa and ataxia appear by the end of the first decade and are gradually progressive. The neurological features are partly due to prolonged vitamin E deficiency. Cardiac arrhythmias can occur and may lead to sudden death. Treatment with vitamin E prevents the development of or progression of eye and nervous diseases (Kane and Havel 1995). Vitamins K, A and D and a low fat diet are also recommended. Medium chain fatty acid can be used as a substitute for other fatty acids.

Case 44

1.   DTPA scan with frusemide
2.   Yes (non-functioning left kidney)

Nuclear medicine studies

	DMSA	DTPA	MAG3
Radionuclide	99mTc-dimercaptosuccinic acid	99mTc-diethylenetriamine penta-acetic acid	99mTc-mercaptoacetyltriglycine
Site of filtration and uptake	Proximal renal tubules	Glomeruli	Proximal convoluted tubules and 10% by glomeruli
Dependency	Functional renal tissue	Depends on uptake and excretion	Functional renal tissue as well as excretion
Indication	Identify ectopic renal tissue, horseshoe kidneys and renal scarring	Obstruction, VUR in children > 18 months of age	Superior to DTPA for obstruction and VUR. Can be used for all ages and well toilet trained child
Radiation	Lower	Higher and less expansive than MAG3	Lower than DTPA
When to do after proven UTI	3 months	6–8 weeks	3 months

Case 45

1. Lead encephalopathy
2. Inappropriate antidiuretic hormone secretion (SIADH)
3. Plasma lead level
   Long bone and abdominal X-ray

Lead poisoning

Pathophysiology
Lead toxicity leads to disturbance of porphyrin synthesis and coproporphyrinuria. It also interferes with the breakdown of RNA by inhibiting pyrimidine 5 nucleotidase, causing the appearance of punctate basophilia. There are also disturbances in carbohydrate metabolism, cell membrane transport and renal tubular absorption. The toxic level at which signs and symptoms may appear varies from child to child. Symptoms are unlikely if the whole blood lead level is < 2.5 μmol/l. Some behaviour problems and learning difficulties can manifest with a lead level between 1.4 and 2.9 μmol/l. Sources of lead poisoning vary from sucking or chewing lead paint to an Indian makeup for the eyes which contains high levels of lead.

Clinical features
Chronic lead poisoning may present with abdominal pain, pallor, anorexia, irritability and failure to thrive. In the acute stage, drowsiness, convulsion and coma may be the initial presentation (encephalopathic picture). Some children can present with intellectual impairment alone. Hypochromic, microcytic anaemia is common with punctate basophilia.

There is increased urinary coproporphyrin and laevulinic acid. On X-ray increased bone density with transverse bands at the end of long bones is seen.

Management
The first measure to be taken is removal of the source of lead poisoning. D-penicillinamine is given in mild cases, 910 mg/kg orally twice a day. In severe poisoning, sodium calcium edetate (EDTA) of 40 mg/kg IV infusion over 1 hour twice a day for 5 days or deep muscle injection of dimercaprol should be given.

Case 46

1. Leptospirosis
2. Stool/blood, urine cultures
   Weil's test (serology)

Leptospirosis (Weil's disease)

Leptospira is transmitted to humans from infected animal urine (rats or other rodents). The organisms migrate to the capillaries and cause microcapillary damage everywhere, leading to muscle pain, renal failure, liver failure, meningitis and rashes. There are different species of Leptospira: the commonest being *L. icterohaemorrhagiae* (rats), *L. canicola* (dogs), *L. pomona* (pigs).

Clinical features
The incubation period varies from a few days to 3 weeks; the disease usually starts with the abrupt onset of fever followed by other features—lethargy, jaundice, rashes, meningism and renal, liver and cardiac failure. There is a pancytopenia with high lymphocyte count in CSF and no organism. The ESR is high. The haemagglutination test is positive in the second week of illness and blood culture is positive in the first week of illness. Urine will be positive after 3 weeks of the illness. Leptospira is sensitive to penicillin; tetracycline for 7 days is also effective. There is a live vaccine stock for prevention for those travelling to endemic areas.

Q fever presents like leptospirosis and can be differentiated by culture. Brucellosis is also transmitted from animal to human and can present with intermittent fever and joint pain. It can affect any organ but most commonly the skeletal, gastrointestinal and respiratory systems. Diagnosis is by finding raised titres for Brucella by agglutination test. It is also sensitive to tetracycline and Septrin.

Case 47

1. Bartter's syndrome
   Cystic fibrosis
   Hyperparathyroidism
   Severe gastro-oesophageal reflux
2. Urinary chloride
3. Bartter's syndrome and sodium chloride (salts)

Anion gap = Na - (Cl + HCO$_3$)

Normal anion gap (10–14) and hypercholeraemia	Increased anion gap (> 14) and normocholeraemia
Diarrhoea, fistula	Increased acid load
Proximal renal tubular acidosis	Organic acidaemia
Distal renal tubular acidosis	Lactic acidosis (primary or secondary)
Drugs (carbonic anhydrase inhibitor)	Ketoacidosis

Bartter's syndrome
This is due to failure of proximal tubule reabsorption of potassium and sodium. It is characterised by hypokalaemic alkalosis, polyuria

and dehydration with hypertrophy of the juxtaglomerular apparatus. The children are constipated with growth failure. There is a hyperaldosteronism secondary to the hypertrophy of the juxtaglomerular apparatus with high renin levels and normal blood pressure.

The treatment of Bartter's syndrome is by prostaglandin inhibitor and potassium supplements.

Other causes of hypokalaemia:
- Pyloric stenosis with low plasma CL, K and positive feeding test
- Chloride syndrome with generalised aminoaciduria, renal tubular acidosis and normal CL level
- Primary and secondary hyperaldosteronism associated with high blood pressure
- Distal RTA with urine pH of > 6.

Case 48

1. Plasma and urine ketones
   Pre- and post-hypoglycaemia insulin level
   Plasma lactate, pyruvate, α-butyric acid, free fatty acids, amino acids
   Urine organic acids
   Abdominal CT scan
2. Nesidioblastosis
   Wiedemann–Beckwith syndrome
   Islet cell adenoma
   Iatrogenic

Hyperinsulinaemia
The normal glucose infusion requirement is 8 mg/kg/min. This glucose infusion should correct hypoglycaemic patients without excess of insulin. The upper limit of peripheral glucose infusion is 12 mg/kg/min; more than that will cause damage to the blood vessels, and the infusion should be given via a central line. The common causes of persistent hypoglycaemia are:

Nesidioblastosis
This is the commonest cause of hyperinsulinaemia in babies and children. There is hyperplasia of the B cells of the pancreas; the condition usually presents with profound resistant hypoglycaemia. The insulin level is high and there is ketonuria due to inhibition of lipolysis by insulin. Abdominal CT or MRI is the diagnostic procedure of choice. Abdominal US is valuable in the absence of CT or MRI. Glucose infusion at the rate of 8–12 mg/kg/min is required until subtotal pancreatectomy can be performed. Diazoxide is helpful to maintain the blood sugar, as are chlorothiazides, steroids and IV glucagon.

Wiedemann–Beckwith syndrome
This usually presents at birth or in the infantile period with hypoglycaemia, macroglossia, hemihypertrophy, omphalocele and transverse ear lobe creases.

Islet cell adenomas
These affect the pancreatic B cells and also present with profound resistant hypoglycaemia. CT or MRI is helpful in diagnosis and surgical treatment is indicated.

Inborn error of metabolism
This is associated with other clinical features and different laboratory findings with a normal insulin level.

Iatrogenic, Munchausen syndrome by proxy
It is important to check the family history to see if anyone is diabetic.

Case 49

1. Familial hereditary angio-oedema
2. C1 esterase inhibitor deficiency
3. IV hydrocortisone and IV antihistamines
   High dependency observation
   Emergency kit with adrenaline, hydrocortisone, and antihistamines to take home
   Genetic counselling

Familial hereditary angio-oedema
The condition is inherited as an autosomal dominant trait and develops late in childhood. There is a deficiency of protein control of C1 esterase inhibitor which leads to localised oedema without urticaria. The oedema occurs spontaneously anywhere in the body. It may cause upper airway obstruction which is life threatening. Patients may present with abdominal pain and can be misdiagnosed as having a surgical problem.

The C4 is persistently low even between the attacks; this is mainly due to massive consumption of this factor. C1NH level is variable, very low on protein or functionally defective in 15% of patients. The management in acute presentations may include fresh frozen plasma after initial resuscitation.

Danazol is the treatment of choice and raises functional C1 esterase inhibitor level sufficiently to prevent attacks. Contraceptive preparations may help in girls in the post-pubertal period.

Case 50

1. Fanconi anaemia
2. Hyperpigmented patches
   Absence of radial bone

3.   Full blood count
     Chromosomal analysis
     DNA breakage study

Fanconi anaemia
Fanconi anaemia is inherited as an autosomal recessive trait; it has a
higher prevalence in males than in females.

Clinical features
This is one of the DNA repair disorders associated with a high risk of
malignancy. It can present in different ways, e.g. with aplastic
anaemia, leukaemia, leukopenia, thrombocytopenia and tumours.
About half of the patients will have hyperpigmented patches, 'cafe-
au-lait' spots, microsomy, microcephaly, thumb anomalies, other
skeletal anomalies, micro-ophthalmia and mental retardation.

Patients often present with low platelets or low WCC before
pancytopenia which always starts mild and then becomes severe. The
red cells are macrocytic, there is raised HbF, and the bone marrow
initially shows areas of hypercellularity which disappear as bone
marrow failure occurs.

Diagnosis and treatment
The diagnosis can be made by identification of breakage, gaps and
rearrangement in the DNA of stimulated lymphocytes. The androgen
oxymetholone is being used to prolong survival; virilisation and
stunting are two major side effects.

The only curative treatment is allogeneic bone marrow transplant.
Preparation for transplant may require irradiation, which patients
with DNA repair defects cannot tolerate. Malignancy will develop
sooner or later in 15% of the patients. Half of these will have myeloid-
type leukaemia and the other half will have liver or other tumours.
Androgens may exacerbate the genetic risk of liver disease.

Case 51

This is the ECG of a 6-year-old boy referred to the outpatient clinic with a heart murmur.

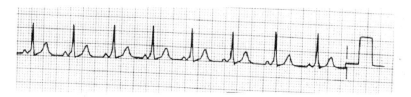

1. What are the three abnormalities shown on this ECG?
2. What is the diagnosis?
3. Name two complications which may arise.

Case 52

A 6-day-old baby has ambiguous genitalia. There is a 2 cm phallus with good corporal tissue, penoscrotal hypospadias, and labio-scrotal folds with a small spherical mobile gonad in the right inguinal canal.

Na	137 mmol/l
K	4.3 mmol/l
C	105 mmol/l
U	4.5 mmol/l
Cr	32 µmol/l
LH	< 0.6 U/l
Chromosomes	45XO (43%)/46XY (57%)
Testosterone	7.5 nmol/l (< 3 nmol/l)
FSH	< 3.0 U/l

Pelvic US—uterus present measuring 32 mm in length, endometrium measures 2.5 mm with short blind vagina. No ovaries were seen.

1. What are the immediate recommendations for management that you would tell the parents?

Case 53

A 2-month-old infant presented to the Emergency Department with a recent onset of lethargy and irritability. She was normally breastfed, although she had received mixed fruit juice on the day of admission as she had been staying with a family friend. She was vomiting intermittently on admission. Her investigation revealed:

Blood glucose	1.3 mmol/l
pH	7.2 kPa
HCO$_3$	12 kPa
U	4.6 mmol/l
Cr	28 µmol/l
Urine	Glycosuria and proteinuria

1. What is the probable diagnosis?
2. What is the inheritance of this condition?
3. What would you advise her parents about her future
   management?

Case 54

A 2-month-old infant presents with a history of occasional wheezing.
At the end of each feed he coughs, but this disappears after alteration
in feeding practice. He is gaining weight but his mother remains
concerned. His chest X-ray reveals right upper zone shadowing.

1. What are three differential diagnoses?
2. Give two investigations to aid the diagnosis?
3. What is the most likely diagnosis?

Case 55

A 3 year old is diagnosed as having a liver abscess. Two months ago
he had a rectal abscess which was treated successfully.

FBC	Normal
LFT	Normal
Anti-B isohaemagglutinin	Present
Neutrophil mobility	Normal
E. coli antibody	High
CH50	33 IU/l (25–45)
IgM and IgG	High with normal IgG subclasses
Abdominal US	Small liver abscess

1. What is the most likely diagnosis?
2. Give one confirmatory test.
3. What is the worst mode of inheritance of this disease?

Case 56

A 2-year-old girl was referred with poor weight gain and a history of
intermittent vomiting. There was no history of diarrhoea or
abdominal pain.

- Abdominal US, CXR, and barium swallow were normal
- pH study excluded gastro-oesophageal reflux

- Urine—no growth of three specimens.

Na	137 mmol/l
K	4.3 mmol/l
CL	118 mmol/l
U	3.9 mmol/l
Cr	41 μmol/l
HCO3	10 mmol/l
pH	7.19
Urine	pH 5.1, no aminoaciduria or glycosuria

1. What is the diagnosis?
2. How can your diagnosis be confirmed ?
3. List four aetiological causes?
4. What is the long-term management?

Case 57

A 2-year-old boy was seen in clinic with a history of persistent systolic murmur. He had suffered repeated chest infections but his parent-held record showed a reasonable pattern of growth and development. Cardiac catheterisation was performed.

	Pressure (mmHg)	O_2 saturation %
RA	5	68
RV		66
PA	33/15 (24)	80
LA	5	96
LV	95/42	95
AO	95/40 (62)	95

1. What is the diagnosis?
2. How would you treat this condition?
3. What are the possible treatment modalities available in the neonatal period?

Case 58

An 11-year-old girl was seen in the Chest Clinic with a history of chronic cough and poor growth development. Lung function tests were performed:

	Pre-salbutamol	Post-salbutamol	Normal values
FVC (ml)	1900	2200	(1950–3400)
FEV_1	1650	2100	(1620–2915)
TLC	2600	2700	(2700–2900)
FEV/FVC%	62	86	

1. What type of lung disease does this girl suffer from based on these results?
2. Give two further investigations of use.

Case 59

A febrile child presented with pain in his legs and back. Weakness of both upper and lower limbs, not previously noted, was found on examination. Ankle reflexes were absent. Sensation was normal. There was no history of trauma. Spinal X-ray was normal.

1. Give two possible diagnoses.
2. What other investigations are indicated?

Case 60

A 7-month-old boy presented with abnormal hypopigmented skin areas on his back and erythematous rashes on the face. Investigations were carried out, including EEG:

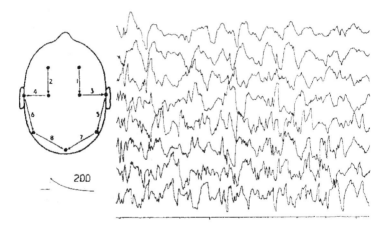

1. Describe the EEG.
2. What is the diagnosis?
3. List three differential diagnoses.
4. What is the treatment?

ANSWERS 51–60

Case 51

1. Short PR interval
   Wide QRS
   Delta waves
2. Wolff–Parkinson–White syndrome
3. Supraventricular tachycardia
   Heart block

Wolff–Parkinson–White syndrome (WPW)

Lower limits of normal PR intervals in infants and children:

≤ 3 years	0.08 s
3–16 years	0.1 s
> 16 years	0.12 s

In Wolff–Parkinson–White syndrome the ECG is characterised by a short PR interval, broad QRS, and delta wave. There is an accessory pathway bypassing the junction tissue and allowing a circuit to be formed which facilitates re-entry tachycardia. This pathway may go from left atrium to left ventricle (type A WPW); this looks like RBBB on ECG. The other pathway may go from right atrium to right ventricle (type B WPW); this looks like LBBB on ECG.

During the attack of paroxysmal SVT the QRS duration is normal.

The prognosis is very good for infants.

Treatment
SVT associated with WPW syndrome can be treated by applying vagal manoeuvres including carotid sinus massage and the diving reflex by applying ice-cold water on the face. This can be very effective in infants. Older children can be treated using either drugs or cardioversion if the child is shocked or not responding to anti-arrhythmic drugs. The drugs used to abort SVT are adenosine and flecainide. Digitalis and verapamil should be avoided as they may cause other arrhythmias. Transcatheter radiofrequency ablation of the accessory pathway can be done if the patient has frequent SVTs and refractory SVTs or suffers from side effects of anti-arrhythmic drugs.

Case 52

1. Registering the child as a girl

Inter sex

The presence of a uterus in this child will make it very easy to make a decision regarding the child's gender. Despite the chromosomal abnormality, the child should be registered as a female. The presence or absence of gonads is difficult to assess. If the gonads are present in the inguinal canal or are intra-abdominal they should be removed. These gonads usually resemble testes and there is no need for them as the chance of malignancy is high. Genitoplasty can be done early rather than late. The parents should be told that the child will be infertile and hormonal supplements will be started at around the age of puberty (12–14 years) in girls.

For the male gender, the presence of the penis is important. 3 injections of testosterone (25 mg) at monthly intervals is a very good test in the neonatal period to exclude the androgen insensitivity syndrome. Children with 5α-reductase deficiency should be raised as a male and genitoplasty should be done early. If the condition is diagnosed later in life at around puberty, then the child should be raised as a female with genitoplasty carried out later (Brook et al).

Case 53

1. Fructose intolerance (fructose-1-diphosphatase deficiency or fructose-1-phosphate aldolase deficiency)
2. Autosomal recessive
3. Avoid foods containing fructose and sucrose
    Avoid long fasting
    Give frequent feeds

Fructose intolerance
The history of lethargy, irritability, sweating and drowsiness is suggestive of hypoglycaemia which could be secondary to a metabolic illness. This does not happen while the baby is on breast milk. In this case the child received for the first time a fruit juice which is rich in fructose.
Fructose intolerance is manifested in three inherited metabolic disorders:

	Fructokinase deficiency	Fructose 1,6 diphosphatase deficiency Fructose 1,6 aldolase deficiency
Inheritance	AR	AR (more common)
Pathophysiology	Blockage of fructose metabolism in liver, kidney, intestine but not in muscle and adipose tissues	Gluconeogenesis impairment in both
Presentation	No symptoms	Late after introduction of fruits in both Hypoglycaemia is the commonest presentation Hepatosplenomegaly

Investigations	Fructosuria Fructokinase deficiency	Fructosuria, hypoglycaemia, Fanconi's syndrome like picture, lactic acidosis Fructose 1,6 aldolase deficiency in white cell or enzyme and fibroblast. Liver biopsy may be required in fructose 1,6 diphosphatase deficiency and enzyme difficult to detect in fibroblasts
Management	Probably nothing Counselling	Genetic counselling and prenatal diagnosis is possible Treatment of acute presentation Life-long fructose-free diet Liver transplant?

Case 54

1. Gastro-oesophageal reflux
    Tracheo-oesophageal fistula
    Hiatus hernia
2. Cine barium swallow
    Bronchoscopy
3. Tracheo-oesophageal fistula

Differential diagnosis in children presenting with vomiting, wheezes, and right upper lobe changes on CXR

	H-type tracheo-oesophageal fistula or laryngeal cleft	Gastro-oesophageal reflux	Hiatus hernia
Clinical features	Vomiting, recurrent aspiration, wheezes	Vomiting, recurrent aspiration, wheezes, failure to thrive	Vomiting on lying down, oesophagitis, occasional aspiration
Investigations	Cine barium swallow, Bronchoscopy ± endoscopy	Barium swallow, pH study, chest X-ray	Barium swallow, upper GIT endoscopy
Management	Surgical repair	Antireflux, consider Nissen's fundoplication in severe cases and children with cerebral palsy	Antireflux and surgical repair if not controlled by antireflux or stenosis develops

Case 55

1. Chronic granulomatous disease (CGD)
2. Nitroblue test (NBT)
3. X-linked recessive

Suggested first line investigations for children suspected of having immune deficiency

Disease	Presentation	Investigations
Hypogammaglobulinaemia IgM, IgA, IgG subclass deficiency Hyper IgE syndrome	Pneumonia, otitis media, osteomyelitis, meningitis	IGs, IgG subclasses, absent thymus, full blood count + differential, CH50
Cellular immunity (e.g. AIDS)	Frequent viral infections, muco-cutaneous candidiasis, PCP	Full blood count + differential, CH50, lymphocyte subset, absent tonsils
Pyridoxase deficiency (chronic granulomatous disease)	Frequent abscess (liver, lung and neck)	Nitroblue test, neutrophil function
Cyclic neutropenia	Skin sepsis and otitis media	Timed white cell count with differential
Complement defect	Respiratory, GIT infections and recurrent meningitis	Defect on alternative pathway or deficiency in terminal component
Immotile cilia syndrome	Pneumonia, sinusitis, bronchiectasis	Bronchoscopy

Case 56

1. Proximal (primary) renal tubular acidosis
2. Ammonia chloride loading test
3. Galactosaemia, Wilson's disease, heavy metal poisoning, e.g. lead, mercury, glycogen storage diseases
4. $NaHCO_3$ (high dose)
   K supplement

Renal tubular acidosis (RTA)

	Distal renal tubular acidosis	Proximal renal tubular acidosis
Proteinuria	No	Yes
Glycosuria	No	Yes
Phosphaturia	No	Yes
Bicarbonaturia	No	Yes
Urine pH	Alkaline	If HCO_3 >16–18 mmol/l, pH > 5.5 If HCO_3 < 16–18 mmol/l, pH < 5.5
Calcium	Increased	Increased
Plasma chloride	Increased	Increased
HCO_3	Low	Low
K	Low	Low
Nephrocalcinosis	Yes	No?
Inheritance	AD/X-linked and sporadic	AR/AD/X-linked and sporadic
Treatment	$NaHCO_3$ (2–5 mmol/ kg/day), K, HCO_3/or citrate if K low	$NaHCO_3$, K, correct acidosis Vitamin D (treat the cause)

Case 57

1. Patent ductus arteriosus
2. Ligation or transvenous umbrella ablation
3. Fluid restriction
   Indomethacin

Patent ductus arteriosus (PDA)

Causes
PDA is commonly associated with maternal rubella infection during early pregnancy. It is also common in premature babies. PDA that persists beyond the first few weeks of life will rarely close spontaneously. In premature babies, if early surgical ligation or pharmacological closure of PDA is not required, spontaneous closure will occur in most of the babies.

Pathophysiology
If the PDA is small then the pressure in the right ventricle and atrium as well as the pulmonary artery is normal. If the PDA is large, pulmonary artery pressure will elevate to the systemic level and may lead to a high risk of developing pulmonary vascular disease. Also a large PDA may cause congestive cardiac failure.

Clinical features
There will be wide pulse pressure and a bounding pulse. The murmur is a machinery murmur heard on the chest in the 2nd intercostal space and on interscapular. A thrill is common, and heart size is normal on chest X-ray. The ECG will show biventricular hypertrophy. On echocardiography the left atrium/aortic ratio is increased and the left atrium/left ventricular dimension is also increased.

A continuous murmur may be heard with the following conditions:

- Aorto-pulmonary window defect
- Valsalva aneurysm
- Coronary arterio-venous fistulas
- Pulmonary artery branch stenosis
- Peripheral arterio-venous fistulas
- VSD and aortic incompetence
- Aortic incompetence and mitral incompetence in rheumatic fever

Management
There is a risk of heart failure and subacute bacterial endocarditis at any age. Pulmonary hypertension is not a contraindication for closure at any age if, at catheterisation, the flow is still predominantly left to right and there is no severe pulmonary vascular disease. New closure techniques besides transvenous umbrella ligation include thoracoscopic surgical ligation; this technique is used in large centres.

Case 58

1. Obstructive lung disease
2. Sweat test
   Immunoglobulin levels
   Bronchoscopy and ciliary function

Restrictive lung disease
The common causes are cystic fibrosis, pulmonary infection, pulmonary oedema, fibrosing alveolitis and neuromuscular disorders.

Obstructive lung disease
The common causes are bronchiolitis, asthma, bronchiectasis and cystic fibrosis.

Lung function
Forced vital capacity (FVC) is the maximum volume of gas that can be expired as forcefully and rapidly as possible after a maximum inspiration. This can be measured in litres per minute by a spirometer. FVC is normally equal to a slow vital capacity (VC). FVC and VC should be within 5% of each other. In obstructive lung disease the FVC is lower than the VC.

Forced expiratory volume in 1 minute (FEV_1) is the volume of gas expired over a given time interval from the beginning of FVC measurement. It is reduced in obstructive lung disease whether it involves small or large airways. In restrictive lung diseases, e.g. cystic fibrosis, fibrosing alveolitis, etc., it is also reduced but remains proportional to FVC. This is not the case in obstructive lung disease, in which FVC is preserved and FEV_1 value is reduced.

FEV_1/FVC ratio is reduced in obstructive lung disease and is normal or high in restrictive lung disease.

Forced expiration flow 25–75% ($FEF_{25-75\%}$) is the average flow during the middle volume of the FVC manoeuvre. The $FEF_{25-75\%}$ may suggest changes in the small airways and should not be used to diagnose the defects in small airways. It is reduced in both restrictive and obstructive lung disease

Case 59

1. Guillain–Barré syndrome
   Spinal tumour
2. Spinal and cranial MRI
   Lumbar puncture if MRI normal
   Nerve conduction study

Differential diagnosis—outcome of lumbar puncture
The history of headache and muscle pain following a viral infection will be difficult to diagnose unless you have done another

investigation. The investigation at this stage will be a CT scan followed by lumbar puncture. The most likely diagnosis is Guillain–Barré syndrome.

A fundal examination or head CT scan prior to lumbar puncture is recommended if there is a suspicious increase in intracranial pressure. Herniation with lumbar puncture occurs in between 4.6 and 6.4% of meningitic patients.

	Glucose (0.66 of blood level)	Protein (0.2–0.4 g/l)	Cells (newborn WCC up to 10 is normal)	Pressure (8–10 mmHg)	Culture
Bacterial meningitis	Low	High	Polymorphs	Normal or increased	Positive in many cases
Viral meningitis	Low or normal	Normal	Lymphocytes	Normal or increased	Negative (PCR helpful)
TB meningitis	Low	High (200 mg/dl)	Lymphocytes	Increased	12–27% positive
Brain abscess	Low in 30%	Normal	Sterile leukocytosis	High—LP contraindicated	Sterile
Tumour	Normal or low	Normal	Sterile (malignant cells)	High—LP contraindicated	Sterile
Guillain–Barré syndrome	Normal	High	Normal	Normal	Sterile
Mycotic meningitis	Low	High	High lymphocytes	Normal	Occasional positive
Encephalitis	Normal	High	Normal or high lymphocytes	High—CT scan indicated	PCR is helpful

In this case CSF will show high protein and normal sugar with low WCC CSF cells. All of these render the diagnosis of Guillain–Barré syndrome most likely.

Myeloencephalitis may present like this at the beginning but focal neurological signs with upper and lower motor tract signs will appear later.

Case 60

1. Very high amplitude slow waves, multifocal asynchronous spikes and sharp waves (hypsarrhythmia)
2. Infantile spasms
3. Tuberous sclerosis
   Infection
   Idiopathic
   Inborn metabolic error
4. ACTH or vigabatrin

Infantile spasms
Infantile spasms are both a type of seizure and a syndrome of multiple causes. The first attack occurs in the first year of life in 90% of cases.

Causes
- Neurocutaneous syndromes, e.g. tuberous sclerosis, neurofibromatosis, Ito syndrome, incontinentia pigmenti, linear naevus and Sturge–Weber syndrome
- Brain malformations, e.g. Aicardi syndrome, agyria-pachygyria, hemimegalencephaly
- Intrauterine infection (CMV)
- Hypoxic ischaemic encephalopathy
- Metabolic diseases, e.g. phenylketonuria, maple syrup urine disease, urea cycle defect, non-ketotic hyperglycinaemia, pyridoxine deficiency, mitochondrial disorders, carbohydrate-deficient glycoprotein and many others
- Other causes—trauma, poisoning, haemorrhage, cardiac surgery and hypothermia.

In 10–14% of cases infantile spasms are cryptogenic; this group has the most favourable diagnosis (Vigevano 1993).

Diagnosis
The attack is a sudden brief flexion of head and trunk, raising of both arms forward, and sometimes elbow flexion and leg flexion at the hips. A detailed history from the mother or father is the key for diagnosis.

The ictal EEG consists of generalised high amplitude slow waves coinciding with clinical activity, with superimposed fast activity. Hypsarrhythmia is a characteristic feature of infantile spasms. It is characterised by the chaotic succession of very high amplitude slow waves, multifocal asynchronous spikes and sharp waves. Neuroimaging and a metabolic screen is essential if no obvious cause is found.

Treatment
ACTH and corticosteroids are most effective. A controlled study between ACTH and corticosteroids did not show any superiority of one product over the other. ACTH doses varied between 20 IU/kg and 150 IU/kg, usually starting with a small dose and increasing slowly.

Hydrocortisone doses are between 10 and 25 mg/kg/day. ACTH and steroids control the spasms in 50–70% as well as normalising the EEG of a smaller proportion. There is about 20–30% relapse (Aicardi 1998).The treatment should continue for 6 weeks; if there is no response titrate slowly and move to the second line of treatment.

Vigabatrin is one of the new anti-epileptic drugs and it gives control of 50–60% of spasms (Chiron et al 1990, Aicardi 1996). It is highly effective in spasms due to tuberous sclerosis and is the drug of choice in these cases. It is usually effective in the first 2 weeks; if it is not effective steroids should be added and vigabatrin withdrawn. Other drugs in use are sodium valproate in high doses 100–200 mg/kg/day, with control of spasms in 40–65%. Nitrazepam is sometimes effective but is less active than steroids.

Treatment should be directed against the cause if it is known.

Case 61

A 10-year-old boy presented with hepatomegaly measuring 4 cm. The blood was described by the laboratory technician as 'turbid plasma'. Father died at the age of 45 years following a heart attack due to coronary heart disease.

Na	124 mmol/l
K	3.0 mmol/l
U	4.1 mmol/l
Cr	24 µmol/l
Glucose	4 mmol/l
Amylase	1100 mmol/l

1. Give two further investigations to aid diagnosis.
2. What is the most likely diagnosis?

Case 62

These are the results of cardiac catheterisation of a 36-hour-old infant with a history of cyanosis and no other abnormality on systemic examination. A full septic screen was subsequently negative.

	Pressure (mmHg)	O$_2$ saturation %
SVC	10	55
IVC	10	72
RA	9	60
RV	80/8	60
LA	3	65
LV	90/7	62
AO		64

1. What is the diagnosis?
2. How may the diagnosis be confirmed?
3. What is your immediate management of this infant prior to surgery?

Case 63

A 2-day-old preterm baby presented with persistent bile-stained vomiting 16 hours post delivery. His birth weight was 2.4 kg, and his weight had fallen further, down to 2.00 kg. Investigations revealed:

Plasma

Na	120 mmol/l
K	3.0 mmol/l
HCO$_3$	35 mmol/l
U	26 µmol/l

Urine

Na	10 mmol/l
K	39 mmol/l
U	280 mmol/l

1. List three abnormalities identified by these investigations.
2. What is the most likely diagnosis?
3. What are the most likely three causes?

Case 64

A 22-month-old boy presented with a history of progressive loss of vision. He initially presented to his GP at 17 months of age because of concerns that he was not able to follow objects. His mother was reassured. He was admitted for further investigations 3 weeks later. CT scan was performed. It revealed a large suprasellar lesion containing areas of calcification.

1. What other clinical test is indicated?
2. What is the most likely diagnosis?
3. List two investigations of benefit.

Case 65

A 3-year-old girl is seen with normal motor developmental skills. She has only 3 words and minimal understanding of words. She can only understand simple commands, e.g. 'bring your bottle'. She shares games and builds a tower of 8 cubes.

1. What is the most likely diagnosis?
2. At what age is her language development?
3. Name three steps of your management plan.

Case 66

A 4-year-old boy is referred. He can walk but not run. He often trips over. He can copy a circle, cross and square. He knows 6 colours and 3-word sentences. He can understand game rules and share them with others.

1. What is the differential diagnosis?
2. What is his gross motor development age?
3. List three investigations to aid diagnosis.

Case 67

This is the composition of milk per 100 ml used by a mother for her 9-month-old daughter.

Protein	1.56 g/l
Fat	3.6 g/l
Na	0.78 mmol
K	1.67 mmol
PO_4	0.87 mmol/l
Ca	1.11 mmol
CHO	7.3 g/l

1. What type of milk is this?
2. What is the difference between this milk and breast milk?

Case 68

A 4-year-old boy presents with epistaxis. In the family history both parents are Greek Cypriots by birth. Haematological investigations revealed:

PTT	110 s (40)
TT	2 min (7)
PT	13 s (14)
Plt	$110 \times 10^9/l$
WCC	$4.2 \times 10^9/l$ (normal differential)
Hb	9 g/dl
Ret	60%

1. What is the diagnosis?
2. What is the inheritance of this condition?

Case 69

A 10-year-old girl with a history of UTI has renal calculus on plain abdominal X-ray and renal ultrasound scan. Urine microscopy reveals:

Protein	+++
WCC	300
RBC	8000

No organism
Culture sterile
Hexagonal crystals

1. What is the most likely diagnosis?
2. What other test will aid diagnosis?
3. List the other features of this underlying condition.

Case 70

A 5-year-old girl is admitted with a history of drowsiness and unsteady gait. She suffered a generalised tonic clonic seizure at home. She had similar episodes at the age of 8 months and 16 months. Her sibling died at the age of 6 months with progressive seizure disorder and failure to thrive. Investigation revealed:

Na	140 mmol/l
K	4.00 mmol/l
U	3.4 µmol/l
Cr	28 mmol/l
Glucose	5.0 mmol/l
Lactate	1.7 mmol/l
LFT	Normal
Ammonia	600 µmol/l

CSF

WCC	1
RBC	< 3
Glucose	3.1
Lactate	< 1
Protein	34 mg/l
Pressure	9 cm/H_2O
EEG	Generalised slow-spike waves

1. What is the most likely diagnosis?
2. What is the inheritance of this disorder?
3. What is the finding on urine microscopy?

ANSWERS 61–70

Case 61

1. Triglycerides plasma level
   Cholesterol plasma level
2. Familial hyperchylomicronaemia

Familial hyperchylomicronaemia (lipoprotein lipase deficiency)
The history of hepatomegaly and turbid plasma indicates a defect in lipid metabolism. This is an autosomal recessive disorder due to protein lipase deficiency; it is characterised by eruptive xanthomata, and abdominal pain occurring later during childhood. It sometimes presents with hepatosplenomegaly and lipaemia reticularis in asymptomatic patients. The plasma is turbid. Triglyceride is high and cholesterol level is also high (3–10 mg/dl). Abdominal pain is an indication of pancreatitis. There is no risk of coronary heart disease in these patients. Medium chain fatty acid (MCT) can be used instead of other fats in food of these patients. The fat requirement should be 2–3 g/24 h.

Case 62

1. Total anomalous pulmonary venous drainage (TAPVD)
2. Echocardiography or MRI
3. Prostaglandin infusion
   Correct acidosis
   Oxygen
   Give diuretics if in heart failure
   Refer for atrial septostomy and cardiac repair

TAPVD (infradiaphragmatic)
All blood returns to the right atrium in this condition. The pulmonary venous blood may enter the RA, SVC, IVC or ductus venosus. The condition is usually associated with ASD.

During the neonatal period and in severe obstruction of pulmonary venous return the infant may present with intermittent cyanosis, tachypnoea and no murmurs. There is another group which can present with congestive heart failure in early life. There will be a large left-to-right shunt and pulmonary hypertension; the child is usually ill. ECG shows right ventricular hypertrophy with a tall R wave in V4R and V1 and a spiked tall P wave in all leads. Chest X-ray will show a 'cottage loaf' or 'figure 8' appearance of the heart. The diagnosis can be made by echocardiography. Cardiac catheterisation can be done prior to surgery or at the time of surgery. This will show that oxygen saturation is equal in RA, RV and LA and LV, and higher in venous blood before entering the heart.

Pulmonary hypertension is common during infancy, and without surgery the prognosis is poor. Acute presentation at birth is an indication to keep the duct open until further surgery is performed or atrial septostomy carried out if the duct is closed.

Case 63

1. Na low
   K low in plasma, high in urine
   High urinary/plasma urea ratio
2. Pre-renal failure secondary to GIT obstruction
3. Peripheral vasodilation, e.g. sepsis
   Hypovolaemia, e.g. diarrhoea, GIT obstruction
   Cardiac failure

Acute prerenal failure

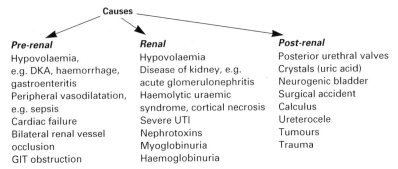

	Pre-renal	Renal
Na (urine)	< 20 mmol/l	> 30 mmol/l
U:P osmolality ratio	> 1:1.5	< 1:1
U:P urea ratio	> 10	< 10
Urine osmolality	> 400	< 400
U:P creatinine ratio	> 20	< 20

Diagnosis
Features of renal failure are oliguria, oedema, acidotic breathing and drowsiness. Acute hypertensive encephalopathy may occur.

Case 64

1. Blood pressure
    Visual fields/acuity
    Fundi examination
2. Craniopharyngioma
3. Urea and electrolytes, glucose, osmolality (urine and plasma)
    Random plasma cortisol, GH, LHRH, TSH
    Head MRI scan

Craniopharyngioma
Craniopharyngioma arises from the remnants of the embryonic Rathke's pouch. These tumours represent about 50% of midline tumours in infancy and childhood (Richmond and Wilson 1980).

Clinical features
These include growth retardation and visual disturbances in children and failure of sexual maturation in adolescents. Bitemporal hemianopia is present in half of patients and homonymous hemianopia in 10–20%. Visual acuity is diminished in one or both eyes in every child (Hoffmann 1977). Unilateral loss of vision may occur rapidly, as in optic neuritis. Focal neurological signs are uncommon. A quarter of cases suffer from hydrocephalus with headache and papilloedema.

Investigations
50% of patients have growth hormone deficiency. Gonadotropic hormones are low in 50% of pubertal patients. TSH and ACTH are less common in non-operated patients but appear in most cases after the operation. Hypothalamic involvement may cause diabetes insipidus or ADH deficiency with lethargy and hypotension. Lateral extension of the tumour may cause third and fifth nerve palsy. Calcification is a frequent and important feature of craniopharyngioma. MRI is the first choice of imaging if available.

Management
Subtotal resection followed by radiotherapy is the usual approach for treatment. Endocrine disturbances are exacerbated with the development of diabetes insipidus in 75% of patients. A variety of psychological deficits are often present. Epilepsy is present in 10–12% of patients. Patients who have not received radiotherapy have a higher IQ than those who have (Pierre-Kahn 1988).

Case 65

1. Comprehension and expressive language delayed
2. 12–15 months
3. Refer to speech therapist
   Portage referral
   Educational psychologist

Suggested approach in a child with developmental delay and no regression

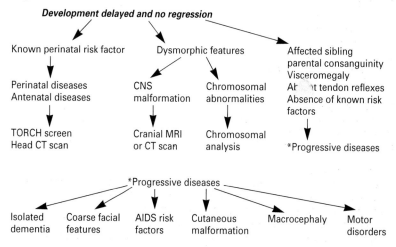

with permission from Gerald M Fenichel (WB Saunders)

Case 66

1. Myopathies
   Cerebral palsy
2. 12–15 months
3. Creatinine kinase
   Electromyography (EMG)
   Brain and muscle MRI

Myopathies
The symptoms of myopathies can be classified as:

- Abnormal gait (toe-walking, waddling, ataxic)
- Easy fatiguability
- Frequent falls
- Slow motor development
- Specific disability with hand grip, climbing stairs, arm elevation, and rising from floor.

The myopathies are characterised by depressed tendon reflexes (not in all myopathies), raised creatinine kinase, normal nerve conduction study and brief, small-amplitude polyphasic motor units on EMG. The muscle biopsy in myopathies is characterised by fibre necrosis, fatty replacement, and excessive collagen. The clinical signs of myopathies can be atrophy or hypertrophy, fasciculations, joint contracture, myotonia and weakness.

Differential diagnosis of neuropathies and myopathies

	Inheritance	CK	EMG	Muscle biopsy
Neuropathy	AR/AD	N/H	Fasciculation, denervation	Group atrophy
Myopathy	AR/AD	H	Brief, small-amplitude polyphasic motor units	Group typing fibre necrosis, fatty and excessive collagen
Myasthenia	AR	N	N	Normal excessive collagen
Inflammatory myopathies	—	N	Fibrillation sharp waves at rest, polyphasic potentials	Peri-fascicular atrophy
Metabolic myopathies	AR	N	Non-specific	Specific enzyme
Endocrine myopathies	AR/AD	N	Non-specific	Non-specific

N: normal; H: high

with permission from Jean Aicardi (MacKeith Press)

Case 67

1. Cow & Gate prem
2. High protein, calcium and phosphorus

Breast and formula feeding

The role of vitamin K and haemorrhagic disease of the newborn in breastfed babies remains unclear. Vitamin K is significantly high in colostrum. The oral supplementation of vitamin K of both baby and mother is having a beneficial effect on vitamin K levels in babies in the early days of life.

Weaning can be initiated at 4–6 months of age but then there are problems of potentiating allergies and causing a deficiency of trace elements, iron, and vitamins.

The food for first stage weaning should contain no added sugar or salt; it should be fairly bland in taste and very smooth in consistency, e.g. pureed fruits and vegetables.

Cow's milk can be introduced by the age of one year as the risk of allergy and iron deficiency will be less. Healthy eating should be introduced as early as 5 years of age.

Various types of milk which can be used in children

Type of milk	Description	Age of introduction	Use
Nytramigen Pregestimil Pepti junior	Protein hydrolysate	Any time after weaning	Whole protein intolerance Milk/lactose intolerance Food allergy
Calogen (LCT) Liquigen (MCT)	Liquid fat emulsion	At any age when needed	Toddler diarrhoea High calorie diet Slowing gastric emptying
Semi-elemental: Nutramigen Pregestimil Pepti junior Peptid 0–2	Elemental based formula	At any age and when needed	Malabsorption states Severe food allergy/ Intolerance
Elemental: Neocate Neocote advance	Elemental based formula	At any age and when needed	Inflammatory bowel disease Protracted diarrhoea
Durocal	Soluble mix fat/ carbohydrate	At any age and when needed	Failure to thrive
Paediasure Nutriprem II	Whey based high fat/protein formula	At any age and when needed	Failure to thrive Children on limited intake
Prejomin	Protein hydrolysate	At any age and when needed	Infant with cystic fibrosis

Case 68

1.   Haemophilia A or B
2.   X-linked recessive

	Haemophilia A	Haemophilia B
Inheritance	X-linked recessive	X-linked recessive
Factors	Factor VIII	Factor IX
	75% reduction in activity and antigen	
	25% reduction in activity and normal antigen	
Severity	< 1% (1 unit/dl) of normal activity (severe)	Factor IX reduction will have same
	1–5% (moderate)	severity as
	6–30% (mild)	haemophilia A
Crossing placenta	No	No
Haemarthrosis	Yes	No
PTT	Prolonged	Prolonged
PT	Normal	Normal
BT	Normal	Normal
Platelets	Normal	Normal
Treatment	25–50 units of factor VIII will raise factor VIII in the recipient to 50–100% (cryoprecipitate)	Fresh frozen plasma Infusion of 100 unit/kg of
	10–15% will develop factor VIII inhibitor. It is essential to continue to give factor VIII in these patients; plasmapheresis is helpful in high levels; immunosuppressive drugs have no value	factor IX is required to raise factor IX to 100%

Case 69

1.   Homocystinuria
2.   Nitroprusside test
3.   Cardiovascular system, central nervous system and eyes

	Homocystinuria	Marfan's syndrome
Inheritance	Autosomal recessive	Autosomal dominant
Enzyme defect	Cystathionine synthetase (type I)	None
	Methyl cobalamin formation (type II)	
	Methylenetetrahydrofolate reductase (type III)	
Ocular	Lens subluxation (up)	Lens subluxation (down)
Skeletal	Tall, thin and long limbs	Same as homocystinuria
	Scoliosis	
	Pectus excavatum	
	Crowded teeth	
	Osteoporosis	

Heart defect	None	Aortic valve regurgitation Mitral valve prolapse
Embolic phenomena	Present	None
Intelligence	50% normal	40–50% normal
Complication	Optic atrophy Cor pulmonale Severe hypertension	
Diagnosis	Increase in urine excretion of methionine and homocystine Low plasma cystine Liver biopsy and cultured fibroblast for enzymatic assay	Normal plasma and urine amino acids Clinical
Treatment	High dose of vitamin B_6 (I) Vitamin B_{12} (II) Vitamin B_6, B_{12}, folic acid and methionine supplement (III)	Valvoplasty Lens replacement

Case 70

1. Urea cycle disorder
2. X-linked recessive
3. Orotic acid crystals

Urea cycle disorder (UCD)
Patients with a urea cycle disorder can present at any time from birth to adulthood with symptoms depending on the degree of the enzyme defect. The hallmark of this condition is hyperammonaemia. A definitive diagnosis can be obtained with the enzymatic assays.

Hyperammonaemia is responsible for causing encephalopathy in these patients. It causes swelling of the astrocytes leading to cerebral oedema and alteration of cerebral blood flow. All of these factors can cause the neurological manifestations in UCD.

Clinical features
Anorexia, vomiting and sleep disturbances in long-standing hyperammonaemia may be due to increased brain uptake of tryptophan and thus increased brain serotonin turnover. The latter may be produced by benzoate, which is used in treatment. The majority of patients present with symptoms during the neonatal period.

Treatment
In the acute form, urgent removal of nitrogen waste products is required. Kidney dialysis with supportive treatment is needed. Later, high protein intake should be avoided and benzoate and phenylacetate used for ammonia disposal. Liver transplant may be the only therapeutic option available for patients with recurrent acute exacerbations of UCD.

Differential diagnosis of causes of hyperammonaemia (Aicardi et al 1998)

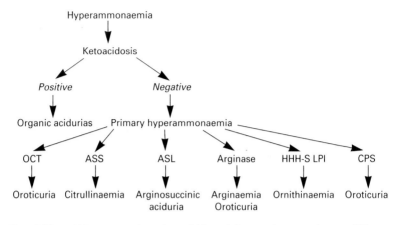

Key. OCT: ornithine transcarbamylase; ASS: arginine succinate synthetase; ASL: arginosuccinate lyase; HHH-S: hyperammonaemia, hyperornithinaemia, homocitrullinuria syndrome; LPI: lysinuric protein intolerance; CPS: carbamyl phosphate synthetase.

with permission from Jean Aicardi (MacKeith Press)

Case 71

This investigation is of a 6-month-old child with a history of vomiting and arching his back during feeding time. His weight is on the 10th centile.

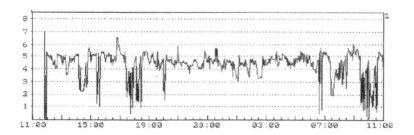

1. What is this investigation?
2. Is it abnormal?

Case 72

A full-term baby was delivered vaginally with a birth weight of 3.750 kg. He was markedly pale and did not feed well. His septic screen was negative. Clotting was normal, as was LFT.

Hb	9.2 g/dl
WCC	$15 \times 10^9/l$
Plt	$166 \times 10^9/l$
CRP	< 5

1. What three investigations are indicated to help diagnosis?
2. What is the most likely diagnosis?

Case 73

An 11-month-old Pakistani boy was referred with jaundice and pallor. His haematological investigations revealed:

Hb	4.3 g/dl
Plt	$260 \times 10^9/l$
WCC	$8 \times 10^9/l$ (normal differential)
Ret	9%
MCV	77 fl
MCHC	25 g/dl
Blood film	no basophilic stippling

1. What is the diagnosis?
2. How may this be confirmed?
3. What is the management?

Case 74

A 6-year-old Caucasian girl presents with abdominal pain. She is lethargic and slightly jaundiced. She has not been ill recently, but a family member has required abdominal surgery for a similar problem. Her results were:

Hb	7 g/dl
MCHC	39 g/dl (34 g/dl)
Ret	13%
Plt	300×10^9/l
WCC	6.4×10^9/l

1. What is the cause of her abdominal pain?
2. What is the most likely diagnosis?
3. List two other useful tests to prove your diagnosis.

Case 75

A 3-year-old boy has a history of failure to thrive. There is no diarrhoea or vomiting. Mother said he does get warm from time to time. She changes his nappy up to 12 times per day. He wakes up crying asking for a drink.

Na	147 mmol/l
K	3.6 mmol/l
U	2.5 mmol/l
Cr	48 μmol/l
Ca	2.56 mmol/l
PO4	1.84 mmol/l
Alb	47 g/l
Alk.ph	278 IU/l
Serum osmolality	292 mosmol/kg
Urine amino acid	Normal
Renal US	Normal
MRI of head	Normal
Serum amino acid	Normal
Urine pH	5.0

1. What is the likely diagnosis?
2. Which other two tests would you do?
3. How will you investigate further?

Case 76

An 11-year-old boy is found to be comatose. His mother suffered a heart attack one year previously.

His blood gases are:

pH	7.07 kPa
PO_2	12 kPa in air
PCO_2	3.5 kPa
HCO_3	14 kPa
BE	−9.3
Urine reducing substance	Positive
Glucose	7.8 mmol/l

1. Describe the blood gas result.
2. What is the underlying diagnosis?

Case 77

A 9-year-old boy was referred with an intermittent history of haematuria and progressive hearing loss. His urinary investigations revealed:

RBCs	++++
Proteinuria	+
Creatinine clearance	Normal

1. What is the most likely diagnosis?
2. What is the inheritance of this condition?
3. What is the prognosis for any affected female sibling?

Case 78

A 9-month-old child can sit alone but is unable to stand. He refuses to give objects on request. He can wave bye-bye and babble. He understands 'No' and will search for a hidden toy.

1. Is there a problem with his development?

Case 79

A term infant was noticed to have extensive bruises over his lower limbs and chest at 8 hours of age. Further investigations showed:

Hb	17.7 g/dl
WCC	11×10^9/l (L 70%)
Plt	14×10^9/l
PTT	60 s (70–90)
PT	14 s (13–16)
TT	7 min

1. What is your differential diagnosis?
2. Give one confirmatory test for each diagnosis.

Case 80

A 4-month-old infant presented with a history of FTT. His liver was 4–5 cm enlarged and he had cardiomegaly. Examination revealed gallop rhythm and engorgement of pedal veins. Investigations showed:

CXR	Haziness of both hilar zones, extending to both lower and upper lobes of lungs
WCC	$10 \times 10^9/l$
Hb	4.9 g/dl
Plt	$300 \times 10^9/l$
MCV	93 fl
Coombs' test	Negative
U	4 mmol/l
Cr	35 μmol/l
Bone marrow	Normal cellularity, reduced normoblasts

1. What is the diagnosis?
2. What is the most likely underlying cause?
3. What is the inheritance of this disease?

ANSWERS 71–80

Case 71

1. pH study
2. Yes

Gastro-oesophageal reflux (GOR)

GOR is characterised by a reflux index of more than 5% at any time during 24 hours' pH monitoring. The presentation is variable and includes: vomiting, failure to thrive, crying during feeding, arching the back during feeding, passing occult blood in stool, anaemia, recurrent wheezes, recurrent right upper lobe consolidation with aspiration, apnoea and coughing.

Prolonged pH monitoring has allowed evaluation of gastro-oesophageal reflux under various conditions. The infant or child needs to be admitted for 24 hours for pH monitoring. If the child is being treated, prokinetics and histamine-2 receptor antagonists are stopped at least 48 hours before recording and antacid and thickening agents the day before. The height of the child is measured and the pH electrode is calibrated using pH 4 and 7.01 buffer solutions. The pH probe is placed in the lower oesophagus using Strobel's formula to calculate naso-oesophageal distance—(height [cm] × 0.252) + 4. Then the probe is withdrawn to 87% of the calculated naso-oesophageal distance and left there for 24 hours. Data is stored on the recorder and analysed with the help of software. It is important that no restrictions are made on activity or play, and the time of feeding, sleeping, walking or playing should be carefully recorded.

Management
For positive proof of gastro-oesophageal reflux, the reflux index should be more than 5% on several occasions; the condition can be classified as mild (5–10%), moderate (11–15%) or severe (16% or above). Antireflux medication can be started: histamine-2 receptor antagonists (ranitidine, cimetidine), a hydrogen pump blocker (omeprazole, not licensed for children under the age of 4 years), and Gaviscon, Carobell or Easy thickening can be used. Cisapride is not used in newborn babies under the age of 3 months and is not recommended in infants under the age of one year. If it is used, ECG (Q-Tc) should be done at least twice a year. Metoclopramide is not recommended in infants and neonates.

Surgical repair (Nissen's fundoplication) should be considered if medical management fails in severe GOR or in a handicapped child with GOR.

Case 72

1. Direct Coombs' test (DCT)
    Kleihauer test
    G6PD level
2. Feto-maternal haemorrhage

Feto-maternal haemorrhage
It is vital to look for evidence of haemolysis in a newborn baby less than 24 hours of age presenting with anaemia. All results can be obtained on the same day apart from G6PD level.

Feto-maternal haemorrhage usually occurs spontaneously in the last trimester with an increased rate during the first and second stages of labour. It may follow amniocentesis, fetal blood sampling, intrauterine transfusion, and external cephalic version. How the fetal red blood cells get into the maternal circulation is still unknown. It can be identified by the Kleihauer test even if only 0.5 ml of fetal blood enters into the maternal circulation.

This test depends on the fetal red blood cells resisting acidification at low pH while adult red blood cells lose their haemoglobin, leaving deeply pigmented fetal cells in a sea of maternal ghost cells. The feto-maternal haemorrhage rarely causes problems to the mother but leaves a newborn baby anaemic.

Case 73

1. β Thalassaemia
2. Hb electrophoresis
3. Regular blood transfusion
    SC desferrioxamine
    Genetic counselling
    Bone marrow transplant

Haemoglobinopathies in children

Thalassaemia minor	HbF 20%, A2 increase
Sickle cell anaemia	HbS deficiency
Sickle cell trait	HbAS
Thalassaemia major	HbF 90% and 10% A2

	Thalassaemia	Sickle cell anaemia
Aetiology	Imbalance in globin chain production	Substitution of valine for glutamine in position 6 of the β chain for HbS
Presentation	Before 1st birthday	After 6 months of age and rarely before 3 months of age
Haemoglobinopathy	*Thalassaemia major: HbF + A2 HbF > 90% HbA2 10% *Thalassaemia trait HbA2 + A1 ± F	Sickle cell anaemia HbS + F Sickle cell trait HbS + A HbC and HbC trait
Inheritance	AR/D	AR
Crises	Haemolytic anaemia Splenomegaly Extramedullary haemopoiesis	Haemolytic Aplastic Sequestration Painful crises (hand–foot syndrome) Infarctions
Treatment	Regular transfusion Desferrioxamine (SC) Bone marrow transplant Folic acid	May need transfusions Regular folic acid Analgesia for crises/hydration Bone marrow transplant

Case 74

1. Splenomegaly
2. Spherocytosis
3. Blood film
   Osmotic fragility test
   Coombs' test
   Abdominal ultrasound

Spherocytosis
Spherocytosis is caused by a red cell membrane defect which causes a loss of surface area, and this is associated with the severity of the spherocytosis. Histochemical analysis shows a cyto-skeletal protein defect in the red cell membrane. The spherotic cell has increased osmotic fragility.

Causes
These include ABO incompatibility, thermal injuries, clostridial septicaemia, and Wilson's disease.

Diagnosis
The fragility test, blood film, and MCV are normal but the reticulocyte count is high and MCHC and bilirubin are increased.

Treatment
Transfusion can be given if Hb < 10 g/dl, reticulocytes > 10% and there is an aplastic crisis with splenomegaly. Splenectomy is carried out when the spleen is causing a lot of abdominal pain with frequent aplastic crises. It is preferable to delay this until the child is over 6 years old if possible. Vaccination against *Haemophilus influenzae*, pneumococcus and meningococcus is indicated in all splenectomy patients.

Laboratory features and possible diagnosis in children with splenomegaly

Spherocytes on blood film, low haemoglobin, family history	Spherocytosis
Low haemoglobin, high HbA2,1	Thalassaemia
Aplastic crises with sickle cells on blood film	Sickle cell anaemia
Anaemia, neutropenia, protozoa on blood film	Malaria, leishmaniasis
Abnormal liver function, positive hepatitis serology, stigmata of chronic hepatic failure, neutropenia, anaemia	Portal hypertension
Large vacuolated cells in bone marrow. Sphingomyelase deficiency in leukocytes or fibroblasts, cherry red spot on retina in 25% of patients	Niemann–Pick disease A &B
Gaucher cells in bone marrow and reticuloendothelial system, β-glucocerebrosidase deficiency in leukocytes and fibroblasts	Gaucher's disease type 1 (bony abnormalities, no CNS involvement) Gaucher's disease type 3 (supranuclear horizontal ophthalmoplegia, CNS involvement)

Case 75

1. Diabetes insipidus (DI)
2. Cranial CT scan or MRI
   Baseline hormonal assay (GH, midnight and morning cortisol and TSH, T4)
3. Water deprivation test

Main characteristic features of diabetes insipidus

	Central DI	Nephrogenic DI
Inheritance	Sporadic	X-linked recessive
Aetiology	Failure of ADH production:	Tubules unresponsive to ADH:
	Idiopathic (familial)	Obstructive uropathy
	Post-traumatic	Potassium depletion
	CNS neoplasia	Hypercalcaemia
	Post-hypophysectomy	Sickle cell anaemia
	Infections—encephalitis,	Chronic renal failure
	meningitis	Drugs—amphotericin,
	Vascular—aneurysm/	tetracycline
	thrombosis	X-linked
Polyuria	Prominent	Mild
Polydipsia	Yes	Yes
Glycosuria	No	No
Fasting plasma osmolality	> 295 mosmol/kg	> 290 mosmol/kg
Urine osmolality with DDVAP	> 800 mosmol/kg	< 200–300 mosmol/kg
Plasma Na	High	High
ADH level	Undetectable	High
Treatment	DDAVP (intranasal, oral, IM)	Indomethacin, chlorothiazides, diet low in sodium and protein

Case 76

1.   Metabolic acidosis with partial respiratory alkalosis
2.   Salicylate poisoning

Salicylate poisoning

The pH is low with normal PO_2 and slightly low PCO_2. This indicates a severe metabolic acidosis with mild respiratory alkalosis.

Pathophysiology

Salicylate is a respiratory stimulant, which leads to hyperventilation and respiratory alkalosis in the beginning. This is followed by metabolic acidosis. K and Na are both lost in urine with the bicarbonate. Despite this the plasma Na and K are normal at this stage. When sufficient K has been lost, an exchange of K with H^+ occurs and the urine becomes acidic. This will cause a reduction of salicylate secretion in the urine. This aciduria occurs in the presence of respiratory alkalosis.

Dehydration, hypokalaemia and progressive accumulation of lactic acid will cause metabolic acidosis. The patient has rapid breathing at this stage because of metabolic acidosis rather than because of respiratory stimulation by salicylate. The patient may develop pulmonary oedema with 10–15% of dehydration. Hypoprothrobinaemia may develop and the patient require regular clotting screens.

Management
Correction of dehydration is very important, as is maintaining the patient's electrolytes. IV or IM vitamin K should be given. Hypo- or hyperglycaemia should be corrected; insulin can be used if necessary. Forced alkaline diuresis can be used in moderate and severe cases. Alkalisation of the urine is the important thing rather than the induction of excessive urine flow. Peritoneal dialysis may be required in severe cases. Counselling is essential; the patient should be referred to a psychiatrist.

Differential diagnosis in cases most commonly presenting with metabolic acidosis (blood tests)

	Blood sugar	Blood pH	Lactate	Ammonia	Ketones
DKA	High	Low	Normal	Normal	High
Organic acidaemia	Low	Low	High	High or normal	High
Salicylate	High or low	High at beginning then low	Normal or low	Normal	Normal
Sepsis	High or low	Low	Low or high	Normal	Low
Lactic acidosis	Low	Low	High	Normal	Normal
Mitochondrial disorders	Normal or low	Low	High	Normal	Normal
Urea cycle defect	Normal	Low	Normal	High	Normal
Hyperglycinaemia	Normal	Normal	Normal	Normal	Normal

Case 77

1. Alport syndrome
2. X-linked dominant
3. Good

Alport syndrome

Presentation
Patients with Alport syndrome mostly present with asymptomatic macroscopic haematuria. Another presentation is with progressive sensorineural hearing loss; 10% have associated eye problems (cataract, macular lesions).

Inheritance
Alport syndrome is inherited as an X-linked dominant, autosomal dominant trait; 20% of patients have no family history. It is more severe in males than females. Males develop end stage renal failure in the second or third decade of life.

Prognosis and management
Females always have normal kidney function but have sensorineural hearing loss and a normal life span. Dialysis and kidney transplant is

the mode of treatment in males. If renal biopsy is done early, it will show only slight changes. Later on, it shows mesangial proliferation and capillary wall thickening which will lead to progressive glomerular sclerosis, total atrophy and fibrosis. All immunological studies are negative.

Management of children with haematuria

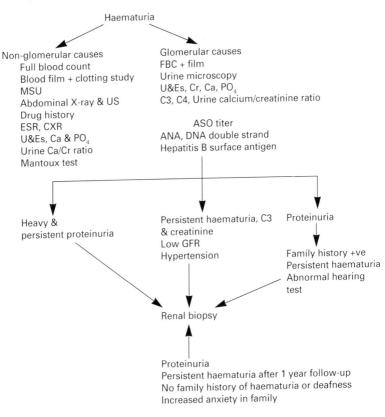

If the family history of haematuria is negative and there is only intermittent haematuria the patient needs reassurance and follow-up after a year. If the patient remains asymptomatic then he/she can be discharged from the clinic, but if there is anxiety and persistent haematuria renal biopsy should be performed as above.

with permission from Dr. Postlethwaite (Butterworth-Heinemann)

Case 78

1.   No. Normal development

Case 79

1. Isoimmune neonatal thrombocytopenia (INT)
   Autoimmune—SLE mother
   ITP
2. Platelets antibody (mother and infant)
   rNP antibody in mother and infant

Isoimmune neonatal thrombocytopenia (INT)   *Alloimmune*

This follows transplacental transfer of maternal specific IgG
antiplatelet antibody from a platelet antigen-negative sensitised   *HPA-1a*
mother. This sensitisation can occur at any time and can affect more
than one newborn from the same mother.

Causes
Chronic maternal idiopathic thrombocytopenia, maternal systemic
lupus erythematosus. Drugs, e.g. isoniazid and sulphonamide, can
produce INT.

Treatment
Options include corticosteroids, which show variable results.
Intravenous immunoglobulins have good results. If platelets are
< 10 × 10⁹/l, this is an indication for exchange transfusion followed by
maternal washed platelets transfusion.

A list of possible causes of neonatal thrombocytopenia
↓

Congenital infection	Full blood count, CRP, blood culture, chest X-ray, TORCH screen

↓ *negative*

Congenital abnormalities (Fanconi anaemia, TAR syndrome)	Forearm X-ray, full blood count, family history

↓ *negative*

Maternal SLE, drug history, pregnancy induced hypertension, IGUR	Mother: double stranded DNA, ANA Infant: anticardiolipin antibodies, ECG

↓ *negative*

Isoimmune neonatal thrombocytopenia	Infant: full blood count, IgG antibodies against mother's platelets Mother and father: platelet count, platelet function and antibodies

Case 80

1. Congestive heart failure
2. Diamond–Blackfan anaemia
3. Autosomal recessive

Pure red cell aplasia

This is characterised by normochromic, normocytic anaemia, reticulocytopenia, normal cellular bone marrow with selective red cell precursor reduction, normal or low white cell count, and normal or high platelet count. The inheritance is unknown.

About 95% of cases occur before 2 years of age; sometimes the condition can occur up to the age of 6 years. The early introduction of steroids is said to reduce the incidence of resistance to therapy. Steroids are usually started with a high dose for 2 weeks then reduced to a very low dose on alternate days. Attempts to stop alternate steroid therapy usually end in success. If there is no response to steroids, regular transfusion with chelation for six days per week is required.

Other causes of pure red cell aplasia:

- Thymoma
- Lymphoid malignancy
- Systemic lupus erythematosus
- Juvenile chronic arthritis
- Viruses—B19 parvovirus, EBV, hepatitis A, B, C, HIV
- Idiopathic
- Pregnancy
- Drugs: anticonvulsants (e.g. carbamazepine, sodium valproate), antibiotics (chloramphenicol, sulfonamide and isoniazid), azathioprine

Case 81

This is an ECG of a 7-year-old boy who presented to the Outpatients Department with a heart murmur. All pulses were palpable and there was a systolic ejection click at the apex.

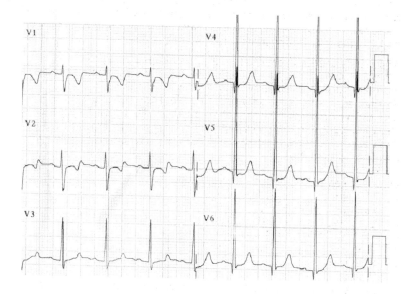

1. What two abnormalities are shown on the ECG?
2. What is the possible diagnosis?
3. Name one further investigation

Case 82

At one hour of age an infant is noted to be dusky and irritable. His weight is 4.7 kg. He is jittery with respiratory rate of 60. Investigations reveal:

Hb	25 g/dl
WCC	15 × 10⁹/l
Plt	400 × 10⁹/l
PCV	77%
CXR	Normal
Arterial pH	7.34
PO_2	11 kPa
PCO_2	4.3 kPa
Be	−4.2

1. What is the underlying problem?
2. List three further investigations to help management.
3. What is your management?

Case 83

A 2½-year-old girl has normal motor developmental skills. She seems to be very shy. She plays alone and has no eye contact with others in the room. She has minimum understanding of verbal words. She can say > 10 single words and no sentences. She plays repetitive games and builds a tower of 7 cubes.

1. What is the most likely diagnosis?
2. At what age is her language development?

Case 84

The following milk preparation was given to a 1-week-old infant.

Protein	3.8 g/100 ml
Fat	3.4 g/100 ml
CHO	4.4 g/100 ml
Na	1.44 mmol/100 ml
K	1.51 mmol/100 ml
Ca	2.8 mmol/100 ml
Phosphate	1.6 mmol/100 ml

1. What type of milk is this?
2. Why is it not suitable for babies of 1 week of age ?

Case 85

At 6 hours of age a male infant born by ELSCS at 31st week of gestation underwent blood sampling. The infant was born after premature labour. Mother had received steroid and tocolytic therapy. There were no respiratory problems and the baby was fed by nasogastric tube.

WCC	50×10^9/l (N 80%, manual differential count)
Hb	15 g/dl
Plt	350×10^9/l

1. What is the abnormality?
2. What is the likely cause?

Case 86

An 8-year-old boy was referred with episodes of abdominal pain and vomiting. The following results were obtained:

Blood pressure	115/70
Abdominal US	Normal
Na	141 mmol/l
K	3.2 mmol/l
Cl	85 mmol/l
U	6.2 mmol/l
Cr	180 μmol/l
HCO_3	34 mmol/l

should be low if Conns ←

He underwent further investigations:

Renin level from left renal vein   6.2 mg/ml/h (1.1–4.1 mg/ml/h)

1. What is the diagnosis?
2. List two further useful investigations.

Case 87

A 15-year-old boy emigrated from India. He has had a history of recurrent abdominal pain for the last year. His father is a doctor and his mother has terminal breast cancer. No abnormality is found on examination. He passes black stools every time he defecates.

Hb	9.3 g/dl
WCC	$6.4 \times 10^9/l$
Na	139 mmol/l
K	4.3 mmol/l
ESR	25 mm/h
CXR	Normal
LFT and clotting	Normal
Abdominal US and X-ray	Normal
MSU	Normal

1. What is the most likely diagnosis?
2. What simple test will you do to support your diagnosis?
3. What is the treatment?

Case 88

A 9-year-old girl presents with a history of progressive loss of vision and painful eyes. She has an area of numbness on her face. Fundoscopy reveals bilateral papilloedema. She becomes ataxic and the MRI shows areas of demyelination in both cerebral hemispheres.

1. What is the most likely diagnosis?
2. List three other investigations of help in confirming the diagnosis.
3. What is the prognosis?
4. What treatments are available for this condition?

Case 89

A 6-month-old girl with a history of seizures is diagnosed as suffering from infantile spasms. She has developmental delay. Examination reveals microcephaly and left facial hemiatrophy with left microphthalmia. There are retinal abnormalities and a dystrophic optic disc. All her reflexes are brisk. Her CT scan shows agenesis of her corpus callosum with grey matter heterotopia.

1. What is the diagnosis and what is the inheritance of this disease?
2. List three useful investigations to aid diagnosis.
3. What is the prognosis?

Case 90

A 15-year-old girl is referred with menorrhagia and anaemia. She suffers frequent bruises during basketball games. Her mother is concerned about excessive loss of blood during her period.

Results reveal:

Hb	9.1 g/dl
MCV	85 fl
WCC	7.2×10^9/l
MCHC	32 g/dl
Plt	350×10^9/l
PT	14 s (14)
KPTT	60 s (40)

1. What is the most likely diagnosis?
2. What other investigations are indicated ?
3. What is the inheritance of this condition?

ANSWERS 81–90

Case 81

1. R on V5 + S on V1 > 35 mV
   Inverted T wave on V5, 6
2. Left ventricular hypertrophy (LVH)
3. Echocardiography

There is increase in R/S ratio on V5 and V6 with decrease in R/S ratio on V4R, V1 and V2.

To assess ventricular hypertrophy:

	Lead V1	Lead V6
Newborn (0–1 month)	R dominant	S dominant
Infant (1–18 months)	R dominant	R dominant
Adult (> 18 months)	S dominant	R dominant

	Right ventricular hypertrophy	Left ventricular hypertrophy
Aetiology	Pulmonary valve disease Tricuspid stenosis TGA Fallot's tetralogy Pulmonary hypertension	Aortic valve disease Mitral regurgitation Coarctation of aorta PDA/VSD High blood pressure Cardiomyopathy
T wave	Upright in V1, V4R	Inverted in V5, V6
Q wave	In V1	In V5, V6 > 4 mV
Axis	Right for age	Left for age
R wave	> 20 mV in V1	> 20 mV in V5, V6
S wave	In V6 is greater than normal: 0–7 days, 14 mV; 1 week to 6 months, 10 mV; 6–12 months 7 mV; > 1 year, 5 mV	Deep in V1 Sum of S in V1 and R in V5 or V6 > 26 mV or > 30 mV if < 1 year of age

Combined ventricular hypertrophy:
Criteria for RVH and LVH
RVH plus inverted T in V6
LVH plus wide or bifid R wave in V4r or V1 over 8 mV.

Case 82

1. Polycythaemia
2. Mother: plasma glucose and vaginal swabs
   Infant: plasma glucose, calcium, U&Es, blood cultures
3. Serial blood glucose
   IV fluids
   Exchange transfusion if arterial PCV > 70% or PCV > 65% and symptomatic

Newborn polycythaemia
Newborn babies with polycythaemia look plethoric; central venous haematocrit is > 0.65 or 0.70 from peripheral venous blood. It is necessary to do an arterial haematocrit if the baby is not symptomatic and Hct > 0.70 from venous blood. If the Hct from the arterial sample is < 0.70 and the child is symptomatic, there is no need to do exchange transfusion. Exchange transfusion should be done with fresh frozen plasma, and Hct should come down to < 50%.

$$\text{The plasma volume required} = \text{estimated blood volume} \times \frac{\text{observed Hct} \times \text{desired Hct}}{\text{observed Hct}}$$

Causes
These include intrauterine hypoxia due to maternal diabetes, pre-eclampsia, maternal smoking, post maturity, and growth retardation. An increase in erythropoietin level in infants with Down's syndrome may cause polycythaemia.

Clinical features

The most common complications in infants with polycythaemia are renal vein thrombosis, bleeding as platelets are low, necrotising enterocolitis, seizures and hyperbilirubinaemia. Infants are usually lethargic, not feeding well, and hypotonic.

Case 83

1. Autism (language and social developmental delay)
2. 15–18 months

Social dysfunction syndromes in children

Social dysfunction of various kinds is the main criteria for autism and Asperger syndrome.

	Autism	Asperger syndrome
Social dysfunction	Deficient in superficial social skills, empathy, compassion	Superficial social skills, empathy, compassion are impaired
IQ	Often low	Often normal or high
Onset	Before age of 30 months	At any age
Social interaction	Impaired (relationship, share, eye to eye contact)	Same as autism
Emotional reciprocity	Impaired	Impaired
Communication	Impaired	Not impaired
Language delay	Delayed	No clinical significant
Imaginative	Delayed	No delay
Ritual behaviour	Yes	Yes
Preoccupation	Yes	Yes
Stereotyped and repetitive motor	Yes	Yes
Mannerisms restricted	Yes	Yes
Cognitive	Delayed	No

Case 84

1. Cow's milk
2. High Na, protein and phosphate

Infant formulas

Casein dominant	Whey dominant
Milumil	Aptamil
Cow & Gate plus	Cow & Gate premium
Farley's second	Farley's first
SMA White	SMA Gold

Whey dominant formula closely mimics the casein:whey ratio of breast milk. There is no difference between the two in terms of calorie content.

Casein dominant formula has a slightly higher content of protein, sodium, potassium, calcium, and phosphorus. Casein dominant formulas have added carbohydrate.

Case 85

1. Neutrophilia
2. Induced steroids given to mother

Neutrophilia
The normal white cell count in newborn babies is $6–16 \times 10^9/l$; 50% are neutrophils. Sometimes WCC can be very high as nucleated red cells are counted and a manual differential should be done.

The causes of neutrophilia in infants and children can be acute or chronic.

Acute (leukaemoid reaction)	Chronic
Physical exercise	Maternal long glucocorticoids in pregnancy (infants)
Response to pain (due to adrenaline level being high)	Chronic inflammation
Sepsis	Chronic anxiety
Systemic mycotic and protozoal infection	Chronic haemolytic anaemia
Hepatic failure	Haemorrhage
Diabetic ketoacidosis	Transfusion reaction
Azotaemia	Post-splenectomy
Bone marrow malignancy	Myeloproliferative disorder
	Leukocytic adhesion deficiency

Case 86

1. Hyperaldosteronism (Conn's disease)
2. Plasma renin activity
   Aldosterone level
   Urinary electrolytes

Conn's disease
The causes are either an aldosterone-producing tumour or adrenal hyperplasia. The excess of corticosteroids will lead to renin suppression and hypokalaemia. Hypertension is the commonest feature of Conn's disease. Hyperaldosteronism is usually a cause of sodium retention; plasma volume expansion, increase in blood pressure and renin suppression will follow.

Conn's disease is very rare during childhood; if it does occur, it is usually due to bilateral adrenal hyperplasia rather than adrenal tumour. Abdominal CT or MRI, or ultrasound will be helpful in diagnosis. Adrenal venous aldosterone level and cortisol sampling may be needed for localisation. Functional study is used to differentiate between hyperplasia and tumour. This can be done by aldosterone response to posture, saline infusion and angiotensin-converting enzyme inhibition. The treatment is surgery for a tumour and spironolactone for hyperplasia.

Case 87

1. Peptic ulcer/gastritis
2. Stool for occult blood
3. Upper GIT endoscopy
4. H_2 receptor antagonist, or
   Na-H channel blocker

Recurrent abdominal pain

This is one of the common paediatric problems occurring in older children and adolescents. The pain is usually non-specific and has been described as colicky, periumbilical discomfort, varying in duration, not radiating or altered by position or daily activity. There are other organic causes which need to be ruled out. Patients with peptic ulceration or gastritis have pain, usually radiating to the back, which wakes them at night, and a strong family history; the condition may be associated with iron deficiency anaemia. Food intolerance may cause recurrent abdominal pain and elimination of certain foodstuffs may help. Migraine may also cause recurrent abdominal pain; there is a family history and response to anti-migraine drugs. Urinary tract infection and renal calculus have to be ruled out. There are also other suggestions that recurrent abdominal pain may be due to alteration in gastrointestinal motility. Constipation can cause this problem, and a full bowel history and examination may exclude it. Abdominal X-ray is helpful but should not be routine.

Other causes which need to be looked for include inflammatory bowel disease, pancreatitis, hepatobiliary disease, and anatomical abnormalities (malrotation, Meckel's diverticulum). Selective laboratory and radiological tests with full history and examination will help to find out what the problem is.

Case 88

1. Multiple sclerosis
2. MRI brain
   CSF for oligoclonal bands
   Visual evoked potentials (VEP), somatosensory evoked response (SSER)
3. Poor
4. ACTH or corticosteroid
   Interferon-beta

Demyelinating disease in children

	Clinical	Neuroimaging	Neurophysiology
Multiple sclerosis	Optic neuritis Sensory disturbances Diplopia Ataxia	Cranial CT may show areas of low density MRI increased signals on T_2 weighted sequence of white matter in both hemispheres	VEP & SSEP increase in latency BSAER decrease in amplitude of wave V Oligoclonal banding present in 85% of patients
Acute demyelinating encephalomyelitis (ADEM)	Multifocal CNS disturbances Drowsiness or coma, seizures	MRI: increased signals on T_2 of both white and grey matter	VEP, SSEP & BSAER are normal Oligoclonal banding is normal
Optic neuritis	Sudden mono- or bilateral visual impairment Neuropapillitis	MRI: increased signals on T_2 of one or both optic nerves	VEP increases in latency SSEP & BSAER is normal Intrathecal IgG oligoclonal production increased
Acute transverse myelitis	History of acute infection in 60% Acute pain and paraplegia Sphincter and sensory disturbances	MRI: increased signals on T_2 of spinal cord	VEP & BSAER are normal NCS is abnormal EMG is normal Meningitis, SLE Vascular abnormalities should be excluded

with permission from Gerald M Fenichel (WB Saunders)

Neuromyelitis optica, Schilder myelinoclastic diffuse sclerosis and AIDS myelopathy are rare in children and should be excluded.

Corticosteroids are effective in the treatment of all demyelinating diseases of childhood; duration and mode of administration vary according to the condition.

Case 89

1.   Aicardi syndrome. It is sporadic
2.   EEG
     ERG, VEP with eye movement study
     Wood's light
     Chromosomal study
3.   Poor

Aicardi syndrome

This is seen only in girls as it is lethal in boys. The clinical features of Aicardi syndrome are absence of the corpus callosum, severe retardation, infantile spasms and other seizures, bilateral choroidoretinopathy with a lacunar (Swiss cheese) appearance, coloboma of the optic disc and microphthalmia, costo-vertebral anomalies in 75%, and microcephaly. Mortality is high because of respiratory infection which is aggravated by kyphoscoliosis. The syndrome is rare. Other associated features are of spastic cerebral palsy or hemiplegic type. Neuronal migration defects, e.g. lissencephaly, pachygyria, and polymicrogyria are often present (Chevri & Aicardi 1986).

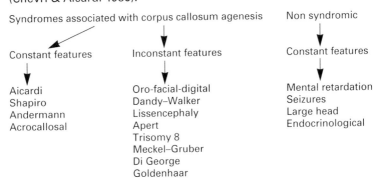

Syndromes associated with corpus callosum agenesis   Non syndromic

Constant features	Inconstant features	Constant features
Aicardi	Oro-facial-digital	Mental retardation
Shapiro	Dandy–Walker	Seizures
Andermann	Lissencephaly	Large head
Acrocallosal	Apert	Endocrinological
	Trisomy 8	
	Meckel–Gruber	
	Di George	
	Goldenhaar	

Ultrasound, CT or MRI scan can be used to diagnose complete agenesis of the corpus callosum. MRI is superior in partial diagnosis. Antenatal diagnosis can be done from about 20 weeks of gestation. The incidence of corpus callosum agenesis is not known; Chung (1974) gives an estimated figure of 1 in 20 000 individuals.

Isolated absence of the corpus callosum may be a coincidental finding if the infant has an ultrasound or CT scan. The child may have normal intelligence or be microcephalic and mentally retarded. In these children, the prognosis is unknown and follow-up is required. The condition may be inherited as an autosomal recessive trait or associated with abnormalities of chromosome 13 and 18.

Case 90

1. Von Willebrand disease
2. VIIIC-Ag, VWF VIII, assay
   Platelet aggregation with ristocetin
   Family study
3. Autosomal dominant

Von Willebrand disease

Von Willebrand disease is inherited as an autosomal dominant trait. It is caused by under-production or dysfunction of von Willebrand protein. There are three types of von Willebrand disease.

	Type I	Type II	Type III
Inheritance	Autosomal dominant	Autosomal dominant	Autosomal recessive
Factor VIII activity	Low	Low	Low
Von Willebrand protein	Low	Normal or low	Low
Von Willebrand function	Low	Normal or low	Low
Von Willebrand structure	Normal	?	Normal
Platelet function	Abnormal	Abnormal	Abnormal

On presentation there is usually a history of prolonged nasal and gum bleeding, and prolonged oozing. The PTT, PT, TT, and platelets are normal.

QUESTIONS 91–100

Case 91

This is a sleep EEG of a 9-year-old girl referred to the Outpatients Department with a history of generalised seizures and abnormal movement of the mouth during the seizure. She had three attacks— all of them at night.

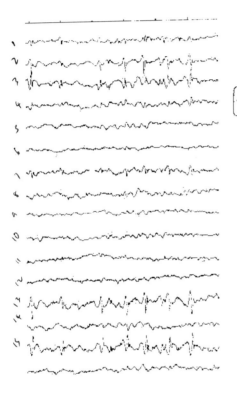 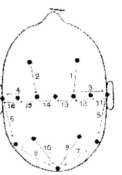

1. What is the diagnosis?
2. What further test can be done?
3. How you will treat this child?

Case 92

This child is diagnosed as having hypothyroidism and a hearing problem.

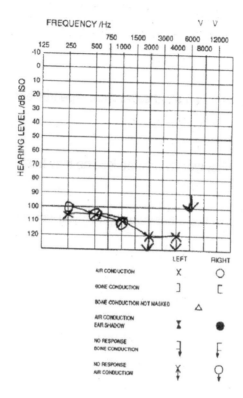

1. What are the abnormalities on audiometry?
2. What is the underlying diagnosis?

Case 93

This is a family tree with a diagnosis of Duchenne muscular dystrophy.

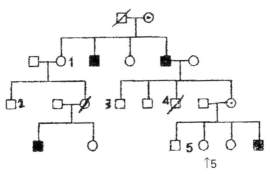

1. What is the mode of inheritance?
2. What is the risk of being affected or a carrier for:
    1.
    2.
    3.
    4.
    5.

Case 94

A 5-year-old boy was referred with a history of nocturnal enuresis which had caused concern for the last 3 months. Recently he had started to suffer daytime enuresis and fecal soiling. On examination, decreased ankle jerks and a reduction in sensitivity over the saddle area were noted. Spinal X-ray was normal and there was no birth mark on his back.

1. At which spine level is the lesion?
2. List three important causes.
3. Name one single investigation of value in this case.

Case 95

A 6-week-old infant was admitted with a history of vomiting following each feed over the last three days.

WCC	$9 \times 10^9/l$
Hb	13.1 g/dl
Plt	$300 \times 10^9/l$
HCO_3	28 mmol/l
Na	138 mmol/l

K	3.0 mmol/l
U	6.6 mmol/l
Cr	45 µmol/l
Cl	85 mmol/l

1. What is the most likely diagnosis?
2. What other investigations are of help in confirming your diagnosis?

Case 96

A 14-year-old girl was admitted with a history of abdominal pain. There was tenderness over the right upper quadrant. A splenectomy was performed at the age of 10 years.

Hb	13.1 g/dl
WCC	$7 \times 10^9/l$
Plt	$210 \times 10^9/l$
Blood film	Spherocytes and anisocytosis

1. What is the most likely cause of her abdominal pain?
2. What is the underlying problem?
3. What is the single most useful investigation?

Case 97

A 20-month-old infant was referred with a history of sudden onset of neurological regression associated with fits. He initially lost his speech. This was rapidly followed by loss of his motor skills. Investigations revealed:

FBC, Mg, Ca, U&E, urate	Normal
White cell enzymes	Normal
EEG	Multifocal epileptiform spikes over both hemispheres
ERG	Flat
Cranial MRI	Marked brain atrophy
VEP	Giant

Vacuolated lymphocytes from bone marrow were absent.

1. What is the diagnosis?
2. What is the differential diagnosis?
3. What are the diagnostic investigations?
4. What is the prognosis?

Case 98

A healthy 11-year-old girl started to have episodes of loss of consciousness. Her colour did not change and her breathing and pulse rate remained normal.

ECG	Normal
BP	Lying 100/70 mmHg, standing 80/60 mmHg

EEG done as part of another investigation:

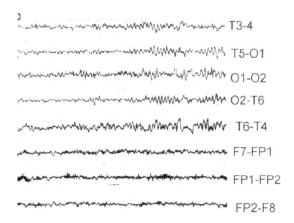

1. Describe the EEG.
2. What is the diagnosis?
3. What is the appropriate management?

Case 99

A 6-month-old male infant presented with watery diarrhoea and nappy rash which had beeen present for the last 2 weeks. The boy was born by normal vaginal delivery and weighed 3.2 kg. The health visitor was concerned that he was failing to thrive. Three uncles died early in childhood.

Hb	13 g/dl
Plt	443×10^9/l
WCC	4.3×10^9/l (N 2.9, L 0.9, M 0.3)
CD3	4%
CD4	3%
CD8	3% (all are low)
PHA	No response
IgG	115 g/l
IgA	7 g/l
IgM	14 g/l
Mg	0.8 mmol/l
Ca	1.7 mmol/l
PhO4	1.2 mmol/l
CXR	Thymic tissue absent

1. What is the most likely diagnosis?
2. What is the inheritance?
3. Name one supportive diagnostic investigation.

Case 100

This is the OFC chart of a 13-month-old boy with normal development.

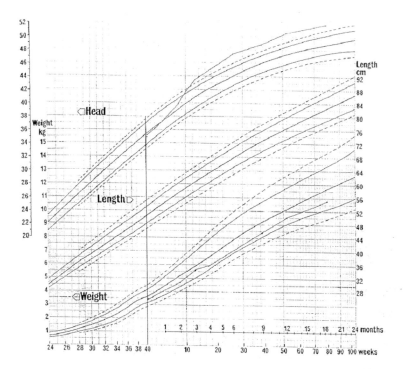

1. What is the most likely diagnosis?
2. What other investigation is necessary?
3. What further steps should be undertaken?

ANSWERS 91–100

Case 91

1. Centro-temporal spike and waves
2. None
3. None (reassurance)

Benign Rolandic seizures
This is one of the commonest forms of epilepsy in childhood, being found in 15–20% of young epileptics. The age of onset

ranges from 3–13 years. About 40% of close relatives have been found to have a history of febrile convulsion, partial or generalised seizures or epileptic discharges in the EEG of a focal or generalised nature.

EEG findings
These include slow, diphasic, high voltage, centro-temporal spikes, activated by sleep. Neuroimaging is normal.

Clinical features
The typical presentation occurs either upon awakening or out of sleep; the child comes to his parents, fully conscious but unable to speak, pointing to his mouth which is drawn to one side, saliva oozing from one corner and often followed by hemifacial twitching. The whole episode lasts for one or two minutes. The other type of nocturnal seizure is characterised by vocal noises with grunting and gurgling sounds coming from the child's mouth, which is drawn to one side and drooling. The patient usually loses consciousness with this type of seizure, and the seizure may become generalised. The third type of presentation is with secondary generalised tonic/clonic seizures. These occur during sleep and last from a few minutes to 30 minutes; they may be followed by a Todd's paralysis (Aicardi 1986). The somatosensory aura is probably common but children rarely report it as the seizures always occur during the night. The seizures usually appear in the first decade of life and disappear in the second. There is no cerebral lesion and the affected child is usually healthy.

Treatment
Treatment is not required unless the episodes happen during the daytime or there is parental concern. Medications include sodium valproate or lamotrigine, but not carbamazepine. About 80% of seizures respond to anticonvulsant therapy. The prognosis is excellent and the EEGs normalise within a few years of the seizures' disappearance.

Case 92

1. Profound sensorineural hearing loss
2. Pendred syndrome

Causes of sensorineural hearing loss
Cases may be isolated or autosomal recessive, dominant and X-linked.

Congenital

Ophthalmological	e.g. Usher's syndrome
Connective tissue	Wardenburg's

Skeletal

Chromosomal

Endocrine

Renal

Neurology

Drugs

Treacher Collins

Turner's

Pendred's

Alport's

Cockayne's

Thalidomide, quinine

Acquired

Perinatal asphyxia

Kernicterus

Aminoglycoside antibiotics

Mumps

Measles

Rubella

Toxoplasma

CMV

Congenital syphilis

Neurofibromatosis

Case 93

1. X-linked recessive
2.

   1. She is an obligatory carrier
   2. 50% chance that he will be affected
   3. Male to male—nil
   4. Male to male—nil
   5. 25% chance that she will be a carrier. The risk has been reduced as mother has four unaffected sons

The daughters of an affected male will all be carriers of an X-linked recessive gene and affected by an X-linked dominant one.

A woman who is a carrier will have 1 in 2 affected sons; half of her daughters will be carriers if the disease is autosomal recessive, and all her daughters will be affected if the disease is X-linked dominant.

Case 94

1. S1–S4
2. Spinal space-occupying lesion (neuroblastoma, sarcoma)
   Spinal dysraphism
   Trauma
3. MRI of spine with contrast

Differential diagnosis of spinal cord injuries

Lesion	Signs
Lesion at level C1–C2	Complete quadriplegia, respiratory paralysis
Lesion at level C5–C6	Quadriplegia, preservation of diaphragmatic movement, sensory level at upper thoracic level with preservation of sensation over lateral aspects of the arm
Lesion at level T12–L1	Paraplegia, sensory level at inguinal folds, loss of sphincter control
Brown-Séquard syndrome *Unilateral lesions*	Unilateral paralysis ipsilateral to affected side, unilateral disturbances of deep sensation, disturbances of position and vibration sense ipsilateral to paralysis Unilateral (contralateral to lesion) disturbances of superficial (pain and thermal) sensation
Spinal hemiplegia *Unilateral lesions*	Either purely motor, respecting the face, or associated with sensory deficits
Central cord lesions	Upper limbs affected > lower limbs, lower motor neurone involvement of upper limbs, disturbances in pain and thermal sensation below the level of the lesion
Anterior spinal syndrome	Paraplegia, loss of pain and thermal sensation, preservation of deep sensation, may be due to anterior spinal artery

Spinal MRI and nerve conduction study are the most reliable diagnostic tests, but a very thorough neurological examination is still the easiest and simplest way to make a diagnosis.

Case 95

1. Hypertrophic pyloric stenosis
2. Abdominal ultrasound
   Plasma pH

Hypertrophic pyloric stenosis
The history is very important in the clinical diagnosis of pyloric stenosis. The child usually presents during the 2nd–4th weeks of life, sometimes later (4th month). The usual story is of projectile vomiting, but not all projectile vomiting is due to pyloric stenosis. A history of vomiting shooting to the other side of the room or dining table is quite suggestive.

The feeding test is very important. Use either the index, middle or ring finger of your left hand to palpate the upper quadrant of the abdomen during feeding. You need to be on your knees on the left side of the infant. This is an important test and is almost diagnostic as it will reveal a pyloric tumour.

Abdominal ultrasound is a complementary test and provides reassurance that the diagnosis is correct. Another criterion is hypochloraemic alkalosis with signs of dehydration. Peristaltic movement can also be observed during feeding, moving from left to right.

Treatment
First, correct dehydration by IV fluid—4% dextrose and 0.45% saline, adding KCI.

Pyloromyotomy (Ramstedt operation) is the surgical treatment. Oral feeding can be started 24 hours after surgery.

Case 96

1. Gall stones
2. Hereditary spherocytosis
3. Abdominal US

Gall stones in children
There are different types of gall stones in the form of cholesterol, bile pigment, calcium and inorganic matrix. About 70% are formed from bile pigment, and these are radio-opaque. Cholesterol is a constituent of 15–20% of gall stones and is radiolucent. Gall stones may present as recurrent abdominal pain and/or acute cholecystitis. Ultrasound is the diagnostic investigation of choice.

Causes and precipitating factors
These include obesity, sickle cell disease, ileal resection and disease, cystic fibrosis, prolonged parenteral nutrition, chemotherapy for childhood cancer and abdominal surgery.

The commonest type of gall stones associated with spherocytosis are those formed by pigmentary bilirubin. They may be formed as early as 4–5 years of age; 50% of splenectomised patients will develop pigmentary gall stones, which are usually asymptomatic. The osmotic fragility test is not done routinely in many hospitals.

Spherocytes undergo lysis more readily than biconcave red blood cells in a hypotonic solution. This tendency becomes greater if the cells are deprived of glucose over 24 hours and incubated at 37°C. A specific protein abnormality can also be established in 80% of the patients with spherocytosis by red cell membrane protein analysis using gel electrophoresis.

Case 97

1. Batten's disease
2. Canavan's disease
    Mitochondrial cytopathy
3. Rectal biopsy
4. Poor

Batten's disease (neuronal ceroid lipofuscinosis—NCL)

NCL is characterised by the storage of certain lipopigments in many tissues. The pigment isolated from normal brain is called lipofuscin, and that from Batten's disease ceroid (Palmer 1989). Lipofuscin normally accumulates in neurons with age, varying in amount, and is regarded as a normal wear and tear substance. Ceroid accumulates in lysosome-like structures. Batten's disease is not, however, classified as a lysosomal disease as there is no lysosomal enzyme deficiency except in the infantile type. The neuronal ceroid lipofuscinoses are not a single disease. There are five types of NCL, almost all of them inherited in an autosomal recessive manner.

Molecular biology diagnosis is possible in types 1 and 3. Antioxidant treatment with vitamins E and C and selenium has been proposed (Santavuori et al 1985). Anticonvulsant treatment is essential (sodium valproate and/or clonazepam). Supportive care for patients and families is very important.

Guidelines for diagnosis of different types of NCL

	Infantile NCL1	Late infantile NCL2	Juvenile NCL3	Late infantile variant NCL5	Adult NCL4
EEG	Vanishing	SW, SIW	SW, SIW	SW, SIW	SW, SIW
ERG	Flat	Flat	Flat	Flat	Normal
VEP	Abolished	Giant	Extinguished	Giant	Normal
Vacuolated lymphocytes	Absent	Absent	Present	Absent	Absent
Neuroimaging	Brain atrophy	Marked brain atrophy	Mild brain atrophy Calcification	Brain atrophy	Brain atrophy
Chromosomal location	Chr 1	—	Chr 16	—	—
Prenatal diagnosis	Yes	Yes	Yes	?	?
Biopsy	Lymphocytes, skin, conjunctiva and rectal biopsy (inclusion bodies). No type of inclusion is completely specific for one form				

SW: spike wave complex; SIW: slow wave; Chr: chromosome; ERG: electroretinography

with permission of Jean Aicardi (MacKeith Press)

Case 98

1. Normal
2. Simple fainting attack (syncope)

Syncope

Pathophysiology
Syncope is a loss of consciousness due to transient reduction in cerebral blood flow. This may be due to alteration of blood volume or distribution, or irregular cardiac rate and rhythm. It is a vasovagal phenomenon causing peripheral pooling of blood. This can be stimulated by the Valsalva manoeuvre, stretching with the neck hyperextended, changing position from sitting to standing, by sudden visceral decompression, or overextension.

Clinical manifestations
Syncope occurs in healthy children, usually around the second decade. It can be described as a dizzy or light-headed episode, or consciousness may be lost without warning. Colour drains from the face and the skin becomes clammy and cold. Consciousness is regained rapidly after a fall on the ground or stiffening of the body with clonic movement of the arms. There may be a period of confusion, but recovery is complete within minutes. It is not a seizure, as a seizure does not produce pallor and cold, clammy skin. Healthy children do not faint while they are sitting or lying down.

Diagnosis
The EEG is normal. Fainting occurring when the child is not standing or arising suggests a cardiac arrhythmia and requires ECG or 24-hour ECG.

Case 99

1. Di George syndrome
2. Unknown
3. Fluorescent in situ hybridisation chromosomal analysis (FISH 22)

Di George syndrome

The data suggest cell-mediated immune deficiency with low lymphocytes, low CDs and absence of the thymus gland. There is also a history of failure to thrive and recurrent chest infection.

Hypocalcaemia due to hypoparathyroidism is another feature. All of these are suggestive of Di George syndrome

Clinical features
These include hypoparathyroidism with convulsions and tetany due to hypocalcaemia, cardiovascular defects mainly affecting the aortic arch, dysmorphic features, e.g. low set ears, microcephaly, and

hypertelorism. Absence of the thymus is associated with recurrent infections because of impaired cell-mediated immunity .

Pathophysiology
Di George syndrome is due to a developmental defect of the third and fourth pharyngeal pouches and the fourth branchial arch. There is a partial monosomy of the proximal long arm of chromosome 22 in 30%, and deletion in 88% as demonstrated by FISH studies (Driscoll 1993). The syndrome can be partial rather than the full picture, because of the heterogeneity of this syndrome.

Management
Treatment of immune deficiency has been successfully achieved using fetal thymus implants or bone marrow transplants (Campbell and McIntosh 1997).

Case 100

1. Familial large head
2. Probably none
3. Follow-up by GP with serial OFC measurement every 3 months

Macrocephaly

Macrocephaly, or large head, means head circumference larger than 2 standard deviations from the normal distribution. About 2% of normal population has macrocephaly, and there is often a familial tendency. Measurement of the head circumference of both parents is important and any family history of large head should be recorded.

In familial macrocephaly, the neurological and mental condition is normal with head circumference greater than the 98th centile. The head circumference may not be large at birth. CT scan will be normal in familial macrocephaly. Ultrasound of the head can be done before the anterior fontanelle closes; this gives a good measurement of the ventricular size. Its diagnostic value is poor for other conditions if there is no familial history of large heads.

Causes
Causes other than hydrocephalus include:

*   Benign subdural effusion
*   Achondroplasia
*   Tumours
*   Giant arachnoid cyst
*   Agenesis of the corpus callosum
*   Increased cerebral volume, e.g. tumours, neurocutaneous syndromes, hemimegalencephaly, cerebral gigantism, Beckwith–Weidemann syndrome, leukodystrophies, GM_2 gangliosidosis, mucopolysaccharidosis and organic aciduria.